The Nurse Practitioner's
First Year
A Guidebook

Shane D Grindle

ISBN: 978-1-913969-67-7

Dedication

This book is dedicated to all the nurse practitioners out there who are struggling to navigate their way in the world of nursing.

Acknowledgment

I would like to offer my sincere gratitude to everyone who helped me in writing this book and making it possible.

About the Author

Shane D Grindle is a professional nurse practitioner who has obtained a master's degree as a family nurse practitioner (FNP). However, being a male nurse, he has had to face lots of difficulties while he struggled to pursue his education and career. Nursing has always been something he was passionate about; he loved the idea of being able to serve humanity while making money out of it.

Throughout his journey, he went through many moments where he was about to give up but did not. The roller coaster had numerous ups and downs and confusions which he believes that not everyone has to go through. This is also one of the reasons why he decided to write this book so that he could share with the world what he learned and the mistakes he made, so the history don't repeat itself.

He wants to share the first-hand knowledge with the world about the things no one talks about. So, if you are thinking to become a nurse practitioner, you have chosen the perfect book to read. Since it is a field that no one feels the need to talk about, Shane decided to bring it to the spotlight.

Preface

As the title of the book suggests, this book is like a bible for those willing to learn about the nurse practitioner as a profession. It talks about the whereabouts and the history of the respective field. I myself being a nurse practitioner aim to share with the world what I learned through mistakes, experiences and how the passage tested every nerve inside my body.

The book talks about the difficulties all nurse practitioners face throughout their journey, especially the first year of the transition from being the student to a real-life nurse practitioner. I also aim to clear the confusion between being a *nurse* and being a *nurse practitioner* because there sure is a difference between the two.

It can be tough, especially being a male, it was not at all easy for me to go after my passion, but I decided not to give up. I am writing this book to share with everyone what it's like to be a nurse practitioner, their first year's difficulties, and how the mind shift of the nurse to the physician can be difficult for many. I am sharing my raw experiences, what I encountered, and what I wished I had known before I got into the field.

The inspiration behind this book is the times of COVID-19, how the profession took a rise and helped deal with the situation in a number of ways. So here's to all the nurse practitioners out there, you are doing a great job! And those willing to learn more about the profession, you are most welcomed to read this book, which is very close to my heart.

Contents

Page Left Blank Intentionally

Chapter 1
Introduction

"I attribute my success to this – I never gave or took any excuse,"

-Florence Nightingale

Nursing school is quite challenging, no doubt, but it pales in comparison to the first year of working as a nurse practitioner. Amateur nurses face many hindrances as they may not have even plumbed while in nursing school. You either manage to quickly secure a position in your dream unit or have trouble obtaining any job itself. The first year for any nurse in the profession is confounding.

Understanding your primary role as a professional nurse practitioner is the beginning of the next phase of the *"rest of your life!"* Isn't that a saying? Without a doubt, this is one of the most exciting moments of your life. With that being said, I venture that there is another place, deep in your stomach, that revolves around the idea of graduation – feeling nervous and curious about future development. This may be because you are not quite sure what it would be like to be a 'real' nurse, and you may not know your working environment. You can develop doubts about your future team members, your own ability to work together, as well as finding the ideal job. You may not really understand the expectations from the new nurse practitioner. You won't know which department or organization you will be employed for, or how it will be different from working as a professional, compared to working as a student.

This guide aims to respond to these concerns with deep insights into how it is like to work as a nurse practitioner and handle the various challenges that come your way. It provides hope and support for you entering the nursing industry. Being able to talk to someone and say, 'Where are you, or I didn't really get this,' or 'Well, this is normal, this is how we do this job' is crucial.

I am worried about all the new graduates operating in a completely independent, effective, and efficient way, instead of stumbling back through the motions. The transition or shift from being a student to a 'real' nurse practitioner is exciting and rewarding. Working as an NP with their ability to control medical treatments can be daunting for many professionals. However, at the same time, it can be fearsome, lonely, and overpowering too. It is especially frightening when the realization begins that you are answerable for what happens with the patients under your care and that you are principally 'on your own.' I like to consider myself as a competent individual. Also, I want to contemplate that I do have some degree of proficiency. In this profession, one transition is never like the other.

You must be mentally prepared for whatever is thrown at you. Moreover, I have expounded my coworkers that, for me, it seems like "whenever it rains, it pours," implicating that when one thing goes wrong, or one patient comes in for others, I get three. Besides, it's almost like harping one's confidence. So, the transition phase from being a student to a real nurse practitioner is the first challenge that a freshly graduated NP experience.

Fresh graduates as nurse practitioners have reported that they felt stressed during their first experience due to the changing role and new work environment. As a qualified nurse practitioner, their pressure comes from the responsibility of being equivalent to a doctor. They also face challenges in managing and prioritizing routine but heavy tasks during the first few months. NPs are required to provide advanced primary and specialty nursing services. A stressful work environment, inadequate employee support, and reduced human resource management departments are the drivers for resignations. These factors also discourage bright young minds from joining the nursing industry. Fresh graduates say that it is challenging to establish relationships with colleagues, which makes them feel rejected by the team. In the first year, fresh nurse practitioners need support from their seniors, as they believe that supporting colleagues can help them adjust to their new role. They are expected to adapt and learn new roles immediately. However, they become frustrated when they fail to meet their or others' expectations.

They also worry about transferring duties and hesitate when they need to communicate with doctors, senior nurses, patients, and relatives. Additionally, when they find a difference between theory and practice in the clinical environment, they become disheartened. Due to the lack of sufficient knowledge, skills, and experience to fill the gap, their clinical performance gets poor. Nursing graduates face many challenges. Also, some studies have found that training, counseling, and mentoring programs can improve job satisfaction, confidence in patient care, and coping with stress. Here, we have identified the following nine areas of care in nursing graduates:

- Workload
- Work environment
- Relationships with colleagues
- Expectations
- Support
- Communication
- Clinical knowledge or skills
- Confidence
- Attitude Issue

Workload

First-year nurse practitioners experience heavy workloads. The acceptable and average ratio of nurse practitioners to patients is 1:12, but most of the time, it exceeds this level and reaches as high as 1:21 in the hospital, but in the clinic, your panel can be as high as 700 patients. A heavy workload comprises doing a lot of paperwork while simultaneously administering multiple tasks. These activities include providing treatment autonomously in ward rounds, responding to the examination of patients and their relatives, offering guidance to student nurse practitioners, and continually observing the administration of dangerous drugs. Heavy workload, lack of manpower, and stretched resources further exacerbate their stress level. As I am in the same profession, I would like to share one example. A nurse practitioner in a rehabilitation hospital must perform all the tasks during office hours. It involves sending specimens because the help section is only open until 5 pm on weekdays. Given the heavy workload, he did not have time to communicate with patients and their relatives, which further caused conflict and misunderstanding. Also, nurse practitioners regularly miss their meals, and they fail to use our break time adequately.

If I talk about the overtime, then 15-90 minutes is quite common in most shifts, and being a salaried employee, you are not compensated for this extra time. Only two out of seven nurse practitioners can cope with the workload, while five of them will admit that heavy workload is one of the primary challenges that affect them. The workload of NPs is expected to increase with the rise of team-based healthcare and primary-care offices adopting the medical-homes practice model.

Lack of Knowledge

Although the knowledge and basic skills learned at school are useful, but they are not sufficient, especially in progressive knowledge and skills. For example, due to a lack of experience and confidence, nurse practitioners experience difficulties in handling emergency situations and transferring cases. They hope to receive basic life support (BLS), advanced cardiovascular life support (ACLS), use of electronic clinical management system (CMS), inpatient drug order input (IPMOE), and other work-based training and blood collection techniques for venipuncture. Many nurse practitioners said that a lack of information was one of the challenges that severely affected them.

The typical responses such as, *"The nurses in the ward are expected to extract the blood when the technicians are off duty, but I was not taught this task in the school." "There are many innovative things in the ward that we did not learn from the books." "Sometimes, I have to assist in clinical procedures that I have never studied before." "The knowledge I learned from nursing school was definitely inadequate for practical use. I have studied many lessons in nursing school, but I have forgotten most of them"* are quite evident that nurse practitioners in the first-year experience that challenges their knowledge.

Communication

During the first year of work, nurse practitioners have difficulty in communicating with different people. Still, the most challenging aspect is dealing with patients and relatives because their expectations exceed what they can provide. This situation quickly leads to conflict. Translating medical terminology into layman terminology can be a challenging task for nurse practitioners. They face difficulties understanding the doctor's handwriting in the treatment record.

However, due to their poor call handling skills, they fear in obtaining clarification from the doctor. NPs prefer to communicate face-to-face with full-time medical staff rather than just reading their notes in the medical record because unprofessional conduct as they want to understand the patient's medical record and medical history to better serve the patient.

Nurses and nurse practitioners can also easily communicate with younger colleagues but must pay more attention to their attitudes when talking to senior colleagues to avoid Whenever they need to transfer the case to a senior nurse, they are under pressure as they fear an explanation with the senior nurses. I heard my coworker saying, "*The most difficult task is translating the medical terms to a layman. It's like translating the English language into Chinese and explaining it to relatives in simple words.*"

Expectations

The doctors, fellow nurse practitioners, family members, and patients expect you to know everything when you are a licensed nurse practitioner.

This category has two expectations, namely self-expectation and others' expectations. Some NPs say that they have high expectations of themselves and others. While several others express that "Expectation" is one of the three significant challenges that affect them. They hope to stick to a precise schedule and complete tasks before handing over. They want to be independent and competent as soon as possible because they do not want their colleagues to be disappointed. They worry about being the object of gossip.

Change of Duty

We cannot impose harm on the patients.

The nurse practitioner's responsibility is greater than that of a registered nurse because they are responsible for all actions and decisions as it relates to the plan of care. In nursing and even nurse practitioner schools, their work is supervised by teachers, physicians, or clinical instructors. As NPs, they must work independently without supervision. All first-year nurse practitioners must follow three working principles; they play safe, take extra time, and avoid hurting the patient.

They were always used to asking their coworkers to double-check all kinds of drug administration with them. Now, they are autonomous being charged to run the plan of care and substantiate many complex diagnoses. Some NPs develop insomnia, which is associated with their responsibilities because they continuously re-think the tasks they handle in the PM shift. They also think about conducting follow-up work in the AM shift the following morning.

Working Environment

If everybody is willing to work as a team, the environment in the ward will improve.

Most of the nurse practitioners establish a good working relationship with their colleagues because of their supportive and helpful nature, and only a few seniors do not intend to provide assistance. A good relationship with coworkers improves the sense of belonging, facilitates self-development in the ward, and augments their motivation and clinical performance. Fresh NPs in the first year feel disheartened when subjected to rumors. They feel bad for being blamed during the handover, which is a common situation in the ward.

Support

The mentor only approached me once but taught me nothing special.

Many supportive programs are offered to the NPs, including residency, orientations, mentorship, and peer support programs. However, these types of support programs vary across hospitals. Residency programs and orientation support are highly effective and beneficial for new graduates due to a lack of real-world training and the need for guided teaching and mentorship. These programs offer guidance in evidence-based care as well as cultivate those novice skills retained during graduate school. NPs need these mentorship or preceptorship programs, as they are useful because the assigned mentors' duty usually differs from theirs. In comparison, a nurse practitioner is a known and respected profession. There are many institutes and universities that offer study and support programs to study this professional line. Whereas, not being offered with these support programs is one of the most significant challenges that a nurse practitioner faces in their first year and dealing with that feeling of not knowing.

They feel frightened and helpless in the beginning. Therefore, they prefer working with their mentor on the same shift. Some hospitals provide a peer support program, which aims to offer psychological support to fresh NPs. Besides, they can have limited usefulness as the mentees are hesitant to disclose personal feelings to a stranger.

Blame/Complaint Culture

Many nurse practitioners mention that a blame/complaint culture is quite common in their workplace. Such culture stems from senior staff, patients, and their relatives. The nurse practitioners hesitate to ask their seniors about uncertainties in work due to their low self-confidence and anxiety. They always think that they would be criticized for their insufficient knowledge. Besides, some nurse practitioners experience criticism by the senior staff over committing minor faults. Such mistakes are merely discrepancies in individual practice. However, they also constitute a significant challenge for first-year NPs.

Attitude Issues

Nurse practitioners are quite optimistic about learning and facing challenges. They learn by regularly searching on the internet, reading books, or seeking help from coworkers or seniors if they encounter any uncertainties. Some of the NPs also attend courses during their personal time. They believe that these approaches will benefit their careers. They may get stressed at the beginning after graduation, but this pressure forces them to read and learn more. This, however, is good for them in terms of their personal growth and self-development. They accept their mistakes and are willing to learn from faults instead of avoiding the same situation. Still, the harsh attitude from the senior staff demotivates them from learning further.

Numerous studies point out that fresh nurse practitioner graduates come across many challenges in their first year after graduation. All these challenges and hindrances impact their psychological health and effect their perseverance about quitting the job.

In addition to the challenges faced by nurse practitioner graduates, I would like to expound on the struggles that you, as a male, might face. My transition from RN to NP was full of a mix of warm and cold experiences. I, too, have faced many problems until I became a nurse practitioner. Some of the reasons why men don't pursue nursing are:

Higher Perceived Expectations

Any NP may struggle to meet the expectations of others. The expectations could come from a relative or a professor. However, being a male NP comes with the additional challenges of facing society's expectations. Since the nursing industry is mostly dominated by females, male NPs have to work much harder only to prove their competency, and even more so to be a capable provider.

Outnumbered

Male nursing students can be easily visible to other classmates and faculty. As a result, they face extra inspection in and outside of the classroom. When you are the only male in the class, sitting quietly in the back of the classroom is not usually practical. However, teachers may still neglect to address the unique problems of male NP students in their curriculum and in some cases, expectations are higher and there is less threshold for errors made by the male.

Treated Differently

Male nurse practitioners are physically stronger than female nurse practitioners and are often asked to assist in lifting critically ill patients. They are more likely to be mistaken for doctors or medical students in a clinical setting. They do not always have the same opportunities as women in the same area. They may lose on the scholarships set up specifically for female students in schools, or they may encounter uncomfortable people, especially female patients in obstetrics and gynecology.

Ridiculed for Being a Male

One of the mains reasons why men do not pursue a career in nursing is that they are ridiculed for being male. Many people don't consider nursing a respectable profession for men. That's why many male NPs experience stress and anxiety in dealing with patients and their families. Sometimes, they face criticism from their own families because of the stigma attached to the nursing profession and the question that always gets asked "So, why didn't you become a doctor?"

How to Break the Barriers

Male nurse practitioners should make a very conscious decision to become an NP. I believe no one should be criticized for wanting to help others. To combat racial and gender biases in the nursing profession, students, nurse practitioners, and other healthcare experts must take the following steps:

- In the school of nursing, teachers, and nurses always have the opportunity to train male nurses. So, they should strive to give them the same attention as other nursing students in the program.

- Female student nurse practitioners should treat male classmates with the same respect, especially in the medical setting.

- Other healthcare professionals should strive to respect males' decisions to become nurse practitioners. The experts should recognize their contribution to nursing and health care and encourage their professional growth.

- Friends and family members of male NP students should avoid prejudice and do not ridicule them over their decision to become nurse practitioners. Instead, friends and family members should support their decisions and provide them with all the help and encouragement necessary to help these people grow personally and professionally. I have been fortunate and had friends that were supportive and proud.

- Patients and their families should strive to recognize and treat male nurse practitioners with appropriate titles and treat them with the same dignity and respect as other professionals. Also, they must provide them with the same learning and development opportunities.

Male nursing students, NPs, and faculty should strive to participate in public events, such as university and career days, health fairs, and/or lectures, to educate the public about the valuable contributions that men make in the nursing industry to showcase and normalize the male contribution to the field. This book will serve as your guide and will help you understand how to deal with the situations after becoming a nurse practitioner. With this book, I want you to know that you are not alone in this roller coaster ride. I want you to know that every other nurse practitioner graduate goes through the same process of adjustment.

I also want you to be patient and recognize that you will go through this experience, and you will become a professional nurse practitioner you have always desired to be. But let's not get too far ahead of ourselves and allow me to tell you how it all began.

A Brief History of Nursing

The earliest professional literature that mentioned nursing was around 300 AD. During this time, the Roman Empire worked hard to establish hospitals in every town under its rule. It led to high demands on nurses and doctors to provide the required medical services. In the Middle Ages, the nursing industry became more prominent in Europe because the Catholic Church promoted healthcare. During this time, many developments and innovations took place, and as we know, these developments eventually formed the basis of modern nursing. The first hospital in Spain was built in the late sixth century to the early seventh century and is located in Merida, Spain. The purpose was to care for anyone who was ill, regardless of race or religion. In the centuries to come, several other hospitals were created. However, their maintenance was ignored until Emperor Charlemagne began to restore them and renew supplies and equipment from the ninth century onward.

In the 10th and 11th centuries, the nursing industry expanded due to changes in European regulations. Hospitals became part of the local monasteries and other religious places. The nurses provided the population with a series of medical services according to their needs, even surpassing traditional medical care. This all-inclusive model is quite popular and continues to be responsible for the various tasks that nurses are responsible for today. In the early 17th century, nursing was rarely mentioned as a profession for various reasons (such as the closure of hospital monasteries). However, in areas where some Catholic churches in Europe remained in the power, hospitals and nurses continued to play a role in the region.

Modern Nursing

Florence Nightingale was a nurse who attended to injured soldiers during the Crimean War of the 1850s. She played an essential role in changing the nature of the nursing profession in the 19th century. During this period, the nurses' role continued to expand because of the need to work on the front line in many wars, where poor hygiene standards often resulted in fatal infections. Nightingale had raised hygiene standards for the wounded in the hospital, which had greatly reduced the number of deaths from infections.

In 1860, with the opening of the first nursing school in London, the nursing profession was further developed. This was the start of many other new nursing schools so that they could receive proper training and education before beginning field internships. However, with more world wars in the 20th century, the demand for nurses increased. The world needed many nurses, which meant that they were often thrown into the field without proper training. Since then, nursing education institutions have continued to expand.

The profession of nursing has also bifurcated out into numerous specializations with further education in specific fields of nursing care, such as oncology or pediatrics. The nursing profession has endured many changes within the last two centuries. The number of nurses following higher education is evidence of the progression of the profession. Many learning options are now available to today's nurses, including the online MSN-FNP program, an excellent opportunity for working nurses.

Let me tell you an essential thing in the history of the infant days of nursing. In the field's early days, nurses were also taught different measures to keep the patients comfortable. They were also instructed about other duties, including laundry, food preparation, and housekeeping. Nurses were also observed as servants of the doctors and were responsible for carrying out orders without ever questioning them.

The speech given to the initial graduating class of nurses by Dr. Hooker at the Springfield Hospital in 1894 specified that nurses must remember that it is the doctor's duty to analyze the patient and that they must refrain from holding an opinion themselves. This is sharply different in comparison to today's standards. Florence Nightingale transformed Nursing Programs to become Science-based. She continued to make incredible progress in nursing education.

She realized the need for formal, continuing nursing education and opened a nursing school in London, the first science-based school, for this purpose. At that time, the nursing industry was primarily confined to learning how to perform basic skills while ignoring scientific intervention. Initially, the industry required a year of training and education, which then increased to two years, and then three years. Nursing was described as a "calling" rather than a career choice, or as a respected member of the healthcare team. As the medical requirements of the civil war were increased, in 1869, the American Medical Association (AMA) encouraged hospitals to implement nurse education programs to increase the supply of trained nurses.

Nursing Licensure was implemented in all existing states by 1921. Slowly, the nursing field began to attract attention as a profession. The demand for healthcare in society was changing and growing. Clearly, nurses were supposed to provide care that met established standards. In 1903, North Carolina was known as the first state to implement a nursing license exam. This proved to be one of the most significant changes in nursing education. By 1921, all 48 existing states had implemented nursing licenses. As medical and nursing knowledge increased, the complexity of patient care began to increase in the coming decades.

Nursing Declared A Respectable Career By The 1950s

In the 1950s, nursing was finally considered a major occupational area. The American Nurses Association (ANA) endorsed that nursing courses require four years of study unless students need only technical skills, which they can gain in a two-year course at a community college. Today, in the 21st century, students must graduate from a college diploma or nursing course to obtain a nursing license, ranging from tertiary to doctoral degrees. ANA still recommends getting a bachelor's degree or higher to practice as a registered nurse, which marks the development of the nursing profession.

The Future of Nursing Education Includes Improved Education

Despite differences among nurses as to the appropriate type and location of nursing education programs, the industry itself flourished in the late 20th century. In the mid-20th century, nurses abandoned their adversarial system of racial and gender segregation and opened equal education, professionalism, and employment opportunities to all nurses. Beginning in the 1960s, new nurses specialized in different hospital environments (such as intensive care units).

Practicing nurses trained to provide a variety of primary healthcare services that began to emerge in the healthcare industry. The emergence of these "trained nurses" enabled hospitals and other healthcare organizations to provide more efficient, cheaper, and safer services. Nowadays, nurse practitioners, clinical nurse specialists, and nurses in other areas of specialization have established themselves. They carry out a large part of all healthcare activities.

Before we move any further with the book, let's examine how the profession of Nurse Practitioner evolved.

A Brief History of Nurse Practitioners

It's been more than 50 years since the profession of Nurse Practitioner (NP) came into existence. You will not be surprised to find out that there are currently 205,000 licensed NPs in the United States. When it comes to meeting healthcare needs, NPs will surely take an even more prominent role in the future. But for now, let's take a step back and look at the history of this humble profession established in the year 1965.

In 1965, Medicaid and Medicare coverage widened their coverage to children, low-income women, people with disabilities, and the elderly. That was about the time when the United States experienced a shortage of available physicians, with an increasing number of new people qualifying for primary care coverage. The NP profession began in response to the scarcity of primary care providers, specifically for children in both rural and urban areas in the United States.

1965 was the year when the first NP program was set up by Loretta Ford, PNP, EdD, FAAN, and Henry Silver, MD, at the University of Colorado. At first, it was designed as a certificate program. Many of the earliest programs were either certificate or postgraduate programs. However, soon in the early 1970s, it became a master's degree program. The NPs primarily worked in pediatrics, but new specialties were created in the 1970s. One of the first family NP programs originated at the University of Washington in 1971, and several adult NP programs began during that same time.

By 1973, the United States was home to more than 65 NP programs. The American Nurses Association (ANA) helped validate the role of NPs by starting the Council of Primary Care Nurse Practitioners in 1974, which also described the initial duties of NPs. In the year 1977, the ANA started offering NP certification exams to further standardize NP responsibilities.

Finally, the American Academy of Nurse Practitioners was established in 1985. Not only this, but the AANP had also accrued 100 members and had begun to develop a national database of NPs by the end of its first year. By 1987, the US federal government began contributing money to NP education, with $100 million spent on various programs. By 1989, almost 90% of NP programs were either a master's degree or a postgraduate program.

However, even as the NP profession continued to grow, NPs did not have provider status in the government's eyes, and thus, they were not eligible for reimbursement. NP leaders worked with the Congress to pass the Omnibus Reconciliation Act of 1989, which, in turn, created limited reimbursement for NPs. During the fiscal health care crisis in the 1990s, many other hospital-based roles suffered. It led to the rapid growth of the NP profession. The number of NPs increased from 40,000 in 1995 to more than 60,000 in 1999. The number of NP education programs continued to outnumber all other specialties.

NPs continued to fight for the legitimization of their profession during the next decade. The Balanced Budget Act of 1997 granted NPs direct reimbursement, and by 2000, NPs were legally able to practice in all 50 states.

The American Association of Colleges of Nursing (AACN) started its lead to require a Doctor of Nursing Practice degree for NPs in 2004. They required that all current NP master's programs transition to DNP programs.

The AACN hoped to reach this goal by 2015, but a document released in October 2014 by the AACN's Task Force on the Implementation of the DNP noted that less than one-fourth of NP programs had fully transitioned to DNP programs.

The number of DNP programs continued to increase, even though the AACN missed its goal of requiring a DNP for all NPs by 2015. There are DNP programs in 49 states, and the DNP is widely recognized as the preferred degree for those pursuing an NP career. The AACN hopes to better standardize curricula, program length, and practice requirements, as more programs continue to transition to the DNP.

As additional patients are covered under the Affordable Care Act, and NPs are granted full practice authority by more states, the role of NPs has become increasingly more significant. Currently, NPs have a full scope of practice in 21 states and the District of Columbia. Moreover, organizations such as AANP are working to increase this number. The NP profession is expected to continue its growth, with 244,000 NPs expected to be practicing by

2025.[1]

A registered nurse's (RN) transition to a nurse practitioner (NP) is a vital career role transition.

This transition is often challenging and can create pressure in different locations. During this time, there is a development from the RN's experience (usually expert) to NP's experience (newbie). It can lead to a change in professional identity, loss of confidence, and weaken the NP role's development. When role development is impaired, it affects the continuity of employment and the decision to remain in the industry. A successful role change is essential to make NPs as useful as possible.

Across the country, the demand for NPs has received increasing attention in recent years. Through the Patient Protection and Affordable Healthcare Act (ACA), the US government directly called for an increase in the number of healthcare providers to care for millions of Americans. They will be eligible for health insurance. Currently, there is a shortage of medical professionals in the United States, and

---

[1] 50 years of the nurse practitioner profession
https://www.clinicaladvisor.com/home/web-exclusives/50-years-of-the-nurse-practitioner-profession/

this situation is expected to increase. NPs are seen as key providers in collaborative efforts to address these healthcare labor needs. However, NP's employment rate is twice that of doctors. Innovative research on transforming the role of NPs has identified many difficulties that they may encounter during this time. Service provider outcomes, such as lower job satisfaction and dissatisfaction, are associated with an increased willingness to leave and produce high turnover rates.

During the NP transition, different personal and environmental factors must be considered to facilitate development. Two of these factors include formal experience and training. I believe no research has been able to directly examine changes in the relationship between NP's roles and experience (exclusively, previous RN experience). There is also a lack of research on finding formal instructions that may help new NPs.

Here, I want to enlighten the readers about changing the role of NPs concerning the RN's prior expertise and receiving precise orientation at the first NP conversion site. Experience is considered necessary for the acquisition and development of skills in medical practice. However, the current situation does not clearly define the knowledge associated with the NP transition from the previous RN experience or with similar roles. According to reports, previous RN experience can provide a foundation and help promote the development of the NP role. In contrast, an NP with less RN experience requires more time to adjust to the new job environment. In nursing, formal induction training is recommended to facilitate the transfer of the role of RNs, clinical nurse specialists, and the NP.

Despite providing extensive training and challenging time for new registered nurses, the NP role still lacks similar measures. In the first year of practice, the lack of structural support will negatively affect defining and educating the NP's role.

This chapter explores whether RN's prior experience is an asset on which new NPs are built. We find whether it is a barrier that requires attention or a combination of both hurdles and assets.

Scope of Practice

During a clinical rotation, NP students are often asked, *"How long have you been a nurse?"* The NPs are asked this question to find if they have relevant prior experience as the RN. Such exposure results in a smoother clinical rotation, and ultimately, a better transition to NP. However, the scope of RN practice is quite different from the NP's scope, allowing even an experienced RN to face a challenging yet exciting transition to a new role. The business scope of RN and NP roles varies according to state laws and nursing committees. RN can develop patient care plans through their unique training to ensure that patients achieve positive outcomes.

These plans are developed through a nursing diagnosis. For example, RNs can diagnose patients with "activity impairment related to pain." In this case of nursing diagnosis, the RN may decide to give painkillers independently before the activity. An RN assesses whether these medications can relieve the patient's pain and reports the findings to the NP or physician to coordinate with RN's pain assessment and develop an alternative care plan.

As NP students learn improved assessment skills to create distinguished medical diagnoses, significant differences appear in the standards of practice between RNs and NPs. With this information, an NP can initiate further laboratory tests, diagnostic studies, and treatment options, including prescription drugs. The NP is also answerable and trained to interpret tests and perform any relevant procedures within their scope business to determine the patient's prognosis autonomously and independently.

Understanding the Transition

The second thing I would discuss here is accepting the transition. Recognizing the difference in scopes of practice between these two positions is crucial to understanding the transformation occurring as an experienced RN becomes an NP. Historically, nurses have always relied on Benner's 'transition theory,' which outlines nurses' transfer of duties from novices to specialists. This theory has been widely expressed in nursing practice, but it does not apply to RN specialists transitioning into new roles.

Benner's theory can be used to assume that the experienced RN has established the foundation as a nurse, and now feels insecure as a novice NP. In particular, this conceptual analysis shows that this high level of instability occurs in the first year of becoming a nurse practitioner.

In a 1997 study, researchers cross-examined 35 RNs-to-NPs after 1, 6, and 12 months after they graduated from a family nurse practitioner (FNP) program and described the stages they experienced. The researchers described the same steps that I faced during my career as Laying the Foundation, Induction, Meeting the Challenge, and Broadening the Perspective.

In the first phase of 'laying the foundation,' the NP has just recently graduated. He or she is seeking a job while studying for the board of directors, obtaining certification, and the ups and downs of browsing through the licensing and certification process. It was the most confusing time of my career. I used to think a lot about making a smooth transition. At this stage, the novice NP lays the foundation for future employment and career opportunities by choosing a professional field and deciding on the best practice placements.

During the 'start-up' phase, NP begins his first job and is primarily concerned about his performance. I believe that the main problem at this moment is the difficult task of managing anxiety, associated with the responsibility of diagnosing and treating patients as new healthcare providers.

Novice NPs may encounter the 'Imposter Phenomenon' at this time, along with anxiety. A fresh NP describes this phenomenon as having the feeling that you are well trained and qualified for the job but also believe that somehow the training is inadequate.

After the first few months of practice, I made different strategies and regained my confidence. These approaches might include a more systematic method for reviewing patient outcomes and treatment.

In the last, I would like to discuss the stages of 'broadening horizons.' Currently, NPs are presented with new challenges and increased involvement in the nursing community's updated practices. This part can be covered by joining workplace committees or national, state, and local NP organizations.

After experiencing the differences between these theories of transition in the practice scopes, I found that even experienced RNs or specialist RNs suffer from confusion when transitioning from RN to NP. The researchers also surveyed around 70 experienced fresh RNs, who converted to fresh NPs and found that the newly practiced NP faced considerably more anxiety during the transition to the new role. In particular, the NPs in this survey felt insecure because they had the responsibility and decision-making ability to diagnose and write the patient's orders, instead of following the RN's role. These NP beginners enlightened that the pressures of the new position were associated with significant nursing changes and that the role of the NP was more focused on dealing with medical diagnosis and corresponding nursing objectives.

Besides describing the transition from experienced RN to NP, I must emphasize the importance of integrating the medical model of nursing with the nursing model of nursing to promote successful role transition. To embed these two different modes of care, experienced RNs should have the skills to use their innate capabilities to organize patient care and employ these existing skills to become leaders in the implementation of NP care.

In a study of 25 knowledgeable ICU RNs, they completed modern practical studies and became NPs. These NPs, who gained a more positive transition experience, can combine their RN experience with contemporary medical expertise. Also, these RNs believe that having an RN experience is a necessary part of a successful transition, not an all-encompassing factor. This case demonstrates the importance of applying prior RN experience to medical models and reminds novice NPs that a confusing factor will persist in the first year of practice when transitioning from an RN to NP.

From the personal records of these experienced RNs, the transition from the RN to the NP is crucial and deserves attention. However, there are still gaps in the factors affecting the development from the RN to the NP. More specifically, I found nothing that supports the view that NP proficiency is directly related to the amount of RN experience. However, most graduate schools require RN experience before enrollment.

Although the RN experience is essential for joining the NP program, some evidence supports this that prior knowledge may initially hinder the new NP transition. I would like to share one case in which 9 RNs, with 0 to 30 years of nursing experience, reported role confusion during the transition to FNP.

These FNPs recall the sensory conflict between the RN's and the NP's, and they often feel that they must return to being confident RNs. As a new NP, with no RN experience, continuing from a bachelor's degree to postgraduate study, one experiences no chaos in any role. Such RNs are free from any doubts and problems in their minds.

Supporting Transition

The research on RN's experience and its impact on the transition to NP is limited. Still, I can elaborate on the general factors associated with the NP role transition. Recent research has found positive results in the smooth transfer of factors, such as the formal guide for the new NP, early identification of role changes at the graduate level, and establishing relationships with mentors.

I believe that the opportunity to experience formal induction training when starting a new job has more impact on the successful transition than having an RN clinical experience. In my career, I have come across people who have received formal induction training. They described a more straightforward transition process and felt more confident and satisfied with the new role.

Now, the Institute of Medicine recommends formal induction training for new or experienced NPs in a changing area of specialization, also known as a change to practice.

Even with these IOM recommendations, there is no universal standard for deploying new practice NPs, and the structure of NP placement varies from organization to organization. I believe it requires more time to understand the direction and training needed for the first year of practice. The objectives for the first working year are to increase confidence, reduce staff turnover, and secure support during the transition period.

In addition to these factors, I also recommend that NP beginners develop personal transfer tools to reduce anxiety, help anticipate and prevent role confusion, and, most importantly, embrace and enjoy the new role. This book will serve as a formal guide for novice NPs, based on my experience on role transfer from RN to NP.

In the last, I would like to provide five guidelines for prospective NPs that can flatten the steep learning curve and increase the knowledge to be proficient as the ARNP.

Understand the Transition

Students should be familiar with the differences in practice scopes between RN and NP roles at an early stage. If something is not included in the practical courses, the student should educate themselves on preliminary research and other previous work on the transition process as an independent learner. The American Association of Nurse Practitioners can be a useful resource for new NPs to learn the scope of practice in different states.

It may also be helpful to collaborate with any available clinical faculty and staff to arrange an NP concealment opportunity to further research and understand the provider's role. NP students may want to spend time reflecting on the changes in the clinical rotation process by weekly talking to clinical teachers to specifically discuss the role shift.

Use Your Experience Carefully

The clinical experience of RN before NP practice can be used in a specific clinical environment. Experienced RNs are quite familiar with how to communicate and treat patients. During a clinical rotation or the student's first experience with the NP, students may feel comfortable and 'intuitive' to continually care for the patients as they do in the role of the RN. Students may be more focused on implementing a specific plan than work as a care and treatment plan operator. Where possible, it may be helpful to learn from the RN's experience in a new job, but NPs must always stay proactive and have a medically driven plan.

Set Realistic Expectations

After many years of clinical experience, RNs should be expected to transfer to a new senior care provider after becoming a registered specialist nurse for many years. Based on my personal experience, NP students should prepare and expect to feel new or inexperienced in this professional field. Students should acquire new knowledge and be aware of uncertainty. They must also embrace the challenges of the learning experience. The transition from RN to NP can last for months or years after the initial certification.

Seek a Formal Orientation

It may be helpful to find employers who will support the NP during this transition period. In the absence of formal guidance, a mentor or designated clinical lead should provide adequate feedback to ensure a successful orientation. The NP anticipates feedback by setting weekly goals to assess achievement and progress upon request. The employer goals and input generated by NP will help maintain expectations of transitional perspectives and ensure active learning and open communication between employers and NPs. All stakeholders must maintain open communication and obtain guidance on expectations and providing a productive working environment.

Find a Mentor

Instructors can help you navigate the elements of work that may not be explained in the textbook or lectures. The mentor can be a moderator, teacher, colleague, or anyone with a detailed understanding of the NP role. The mentor must have gone through the same transition and should provide personal insights into the subject. Combining multiple mentors allows the NP to have a variety of perspectives during the transition to further practice.

Pick Your Employer Carefully

One research observed that novice nurse practitioners were more likely to have a negative experience in the first year if they worked in a company that did not appreciate their role. The lack of preparation for incorporating NPs into medical settings is a stern hurdle. The lack of orientation, infrastructure, leadership, and awareness of the NP role and needs make this transition quite challenging.

One-third of NPs leave their job because of professional conflict with coworkers who do not accept their role and expertise. You must carefully choose your first employer. Make sure they provide new nurses with a supportive environment that meets their professional expectations. Ensure that your first employer knows what a nurse is, and you can be clear about the scope of your practice. Your first year is about teaching, growing, and caring for patients, not letting your employer join a nursing practice. If your employer does not understand practicing nurses, you may be involved in registered nurse (RN) related skills. Employers should not expect you to play the role of a registered nurse and nurse practitioner at the same time. Each designation has its own business scope and expertise. When taking up your first job, make sure your employer understands this difference and supports your transition.

At this point, make sure you understand that this is also a different job. As a practicing nurse practitioner, you have more autonomy, and therefore, more responsibility. Now, these are your patients, and you must diagnose and treat them while leading the medical team. Your higher education and strict certification have earned you the title of the nurse practitioner. Embrace it!

Don't Forget Your Reason to Join

In the first year, you will feel stressed, confused, and tired. To remove this concern, reflect on your skills and qualifications. Remember, you are transforming, so everything will not go smoothly. Focus on what you've learned and never forget why you became a nurse practitioner in the first place. I have mentioned above about the 'Imposter Syndrome.' It is a phenomenon that makes you feel that you are not qualified for the job, and in some way, it deceives and convinces everyone. After transferring from RN to NP, this is very common. The strange thing about this phenomenon is that it happens to people who are actually highly qualified and competent.

I will tell you a secret. In my first year, I was quite nervous! I used to work in an extensive hospital system, operating on different floors and caring for various patients with severe illnesses. Besides, I also had feelings of imposter syndrome.

But my weapon was a piece of paper, which I used to keep in my lab coat pocket. In that paper, I listed the reasons why

I decided to pursue this field. In those challenging days, I used to take it out between the visits and remember why I was there.

Do More Than Clinical Work

Becoming a professional nurse practitioner is not an easy task. However, in the first year, don't forget other areas of medicine that interest you, such as research, technology, policy, and leadership. You are not limited to patient care. Besides, you must make sure you have a variety of tasks.

Get Involved

Don't isolate yourself! Participate in nursing practices. First, join the American Association of Nurse Practitioners. They are a one-stop-shop that provides you with everything that a new nurse practitioner requires. They offer mentoring opportunities, continuing education, social activities, and professional publicity. It's also essential to join a local organization, so you can keep in touch with nurse practitioners living nearby. Joining the community of similar professionals can reduce anxiety during the transition and keep you in touch with others who may be experiencing the same problems.

I want you to comprehend how imperative it is to recognize and prepare for this transition through this book. The new-to-practice NP, who is ready to embrace the trials during the RN-to-NP transition, will be able to navigate his or her new career successfully with my help. This recognition will improve the NP's performance on the job and extend to improvements in patient care.

Chapter 2
What's Next After I Pass Boards?

Congratulations on graduating from the nurse practitioner's school! After years of hard work and effort, you should find a fascinating and exciting job that fits your personality and skills. However, finding suitable opportunities as a nurse practitioner can be onerous as a new graduate. The job hunt and licensing procedures come with a lot of trials. To make sure you are satisfied with your first decision, take some time to understand the opportunities that best suit your professional goals.

Here, I would like to talk a little about my own experience. Being placed in the cardiac transplant unit at one of the best hospitals in the world helped to expound many of my skills gained from being in nursing school. It helped me to hone my critical thinking skills in ways that prepared me to be a nurse practitioner. I was trained with the best physicians and nurse practitioners in the country, and that came with high expectations. I didn't want to let anyone down. So, I sought out positions on various committees, participated in grand rounds, and attended all professional development workshops to be involved and become a well-educated healthcare provider. I was fortunate to meet many great patients that were awaiting transplant and grew close to them. I shared many of their triumphs as well as any lows they experienced with them and their families.

Education was a large part of the discharge process of the patients, and I grew to love education and decided to take up teaching part-time after graduate school. I grew to love and respect the field of cardiology, and I feel that this knowledge is crucial due to heart disease being the number one killer of Americans. It allows me to do my part to prevent this pandemic by educating patients and treating them as a cardio-centric nurse practitioner and referring to the ever-changing guidelines of the American Heart Association.

Anyway, finding out how to land your first job and leave nursing school can be daunting. I always encourage new graduates to look for their careers as strategically as possible.

Here are some stress-free ways to find the best nursing job as a new graduate:

Understand Your Options

Discovering a reputable hospital is usually the primary goal of many NP graduates who want to start a career. However, recent NP graduates mistakenly think that joining a hospital is their only option. I would suggest that there are several medical settings to consider. Such medical facilities include home care, long-term care, and even clinics as potential workplaces. On the other hand, if you are not familiar with the recruitment facilities, consider using the major executive committees. You can explore Indeed or LinkedIn to better understand what the employer is looking for in the candidates based on your experience.

Use Your Network And Resources

Since you can't rely on years of professional experience, using your resources and network are your next best available options. For instance, your care plan may be associated with multiple hospitals, or your assistant professor may be a nurse practitioner at a local institution who you can contact for placement advice. I have observed that many nursing graduates do not consider the school network and different employment types before deciding their first job. If your immediate network or system can't provide a solution, consider working with recruiters. They can link you to work day-to-day or contract jobs before finding a longer-term position. This way, you have the opportunity to see the job environment that best suits your needs and skills.

Get Certified In Multiple States

As a nurse practitioner, you always desire to find a way to stand out from the competition throughout the job-hunting process. One of the best ways is to ensure that your certificate can be used in multiple states. In simpler words, if you are ready to commute and relocate, you must try getting a license in the neighboring states. For instance, if you live in New York, you might want to consider getting a license to practice in states like New Jersey or Connecticut. Traveling to these states is quite comfortable. The additional certification makes you a more deserving candidate in the market, and it can also unquestionably speed up your recruitment process.

Perfect Your Resume And Interview Preparation

The first thing new NP graduates should do before starting a job search is to perfect their resume. This requires checking for syntax and grammatical errors in it. Also, you should get friends or relatives to read your resume and find if there are any mistakes or missing information. Your resume should also include language proficiencies, volunteer work, organizational memberships, certifications, and rotation availability in addition to your education and experience. Consider preparing answers to common interview questions while preparing a perfect resume. Finally, you must ensure that you are fully equipped once you are called for the interview.

The Credentialing Process

The credentialing process of an NP includes the verification of education, certification, licensure, and other references. To be entitled to bill insurance companies and government agencies, nurse practitioners (NP) or physician assistants must obtain their certificates. The initial credentialing includes plenty of paperwork.

In most cases, the practicing manager will help you sort out the process. If you are fortunate enough, they will only mark the pages you need to sign. The typical credentialing process consists of forms, standardized procedures, and agreements to be implemented by the provider. Besides, license verification, copy of the DEA certificate, professional reference materials, etc., are part of the credentialing process. The nurse practitioner (or their full-time office manager) is responsible for collecting the necessary documents and delivering them to each institution.

After the verification of references and completion of the background checks, the NP can start working. Some hospitals or clinics may require nurse practitioners and physician assistants to complete a probationary period. In addition to the process, NPs must conduct a chart review or attend other training events.

When you start a new position as a Nurse Practitioner, be conscious that your credentialing process is in order. It may take a month or two, or even more, for you to begin working. Having your certifications and other credentials after completing the obligatory paperwork will help accelerate the process. It would ensure that you will get your first paycheck on time. You are about to graduate from (or already have) the Nurse Practitioner Program, and I am sure you are feeling ecstatic! But what are the next steps you take from here? The NP certification process can be staggering. I remember, after I graduated, all I wanted was an easy-to-follow guide to simplify the steps. I have found that the exact circumstances may vary from state to state, but the general steps remain the same. Apprehend the steps below to get a Nursing License and start practicing efficiently and successfully.

NP Credentialing Process: Apply for Certification

The road to becoming a nurse practitioner is long. If you are like me, you may be too focused on research and unable to find the precise steps to take after graduation. To apply for a state license, you must first prove your capability to appear in the certification exam. You can appear in the exam through the American Academy of Nurse Practitioners (AANP) or the American Nurses Accreditation Center (ANCC).

The AANP offers exams for the Adult-Gerontology Primary Care Nurse Practitioner (A-GNP), Family Nurse Practitioner (FNP), and the Emergency Nurse Practitioner (ENP). In contrast, ANCC offers exams for the Adult-Gerontology. It also provides exams of Psychiatric-Mental Health NP (PMHNP), Pediatric NP (PNP), and Adult-Gero Acute NP.

For this purpose, you have to create an account and apply for a certification exam within your respective major. The cost of certification from these agencies is reasonably high – the AANP costs around **$315** for the initial certification, or around **$240**. Besides, you will get a discount of **$75** if you are a member of AANP. For the ANCC certifications, non-members pay around **$395**, but discounted prices for AANP members are **$340**. Also, the price for AANP Student members is **$290**, and **$270** for ANA members.

Your educational information is required as the initial certification application demands you to record the details of all the courses you have attended. You will also need to list the name and address of your clinical site. Also, the process requires contact information.

Send Verification Information

The next step in the NP certification process is verification. In case you apply through the AANP or the ANCC, you will have to verify that you are a student of the final semester or that you have already graduated from the nursing school. For this, you must send an official transcript signifying that you have graduated from a recognized nursing program to the verifying bodies (AANP or ANCC). This process has become effortless. Now, you can get this job done through your university's online portal. Many universities provide the facility of fast email delivery, generally against a small fee.

You may still apply even if you haven't graduated or completed school. For this, you must send an official transcript of your work-to-date. It will permit you to sit in the exam, but you need to resend the official transcript after your conferral date to corroborate that you have successfully graduated.

Drop An Email To The Mentioned Addresses

ANCC, Email: aprnvalidation@ana.org

ANCC Mail: ANCC PO Box 8785, Silver Spring, MD 20907-8785

AANP Email: Certification@aanpcert.org

AANP Transcripts Email: Transcripts@aanpcert.org

AANP Mail: AANPCB, P.O. Box 12926, Austin, TX 78711

You will receive an email from the certification body each week to update the required documents. The average processing time is 3-6 weeks. For the ANCC, you can use the "Quick Review Procedure" to shorten the processing time to five working days, but it will cost an additional $ 200.

Take the Exam

Upon successful completion of receiving and processing of all information, AANP or ANCC will send an 'Authorization / Test Qualification' email. In this communication, they will provide you with instructions about the registration exam's venue and date. You will take the test at the examination center – comparable to the one you may have taken your NCLEX-RN at. Make sure to bring **two types of IDs**, one must be your photo ID, and the other one can be a credit/debit card with a signature on it. Most importantly, make sure to reach the examination center at least 30 minutes before the actual time.

The AANP exam has 150 questions, and you will have 180 minutes to submit your answers. While the ANCC exam has 200 questions, and you will be given 240 minutes to provide your answers.

After submitting the solutions, you must immediately conduct a quick survey. You will leave the room upon completion of the review, and the testing proctors for the test will provide you with printed information. Based on this information, you get preliminary results — that hopefully say, "You've passed."

Wait for Official Certification

After sitting for the exam, you will have to wait for the official score. These will be emailed, but they will also be updated on the certification website, so be cautious. This process usually takes 2-3 weeks. Once formally certified, you can begin applying for a state BON license as a nurse practitioner.

Apply for Licensure with the State BON

This stage in the Nurse Practitioner Credentialing Process varies from state to state. You can explore the official website of the 'Nurse practitioner license,' and you will most probably find the BON section of your state. It may have the application form in pdf format for you to download, or perhaps, you have to request an initial certification application through a secure email. Once you have the PDF, you can use any application to fill the form. Also, you can print the form and fill it in by hand. Please ensure to fill in all sections correctly. If there is anything wrong, your permission for the license may be delayed.

Requirements Vary From State To State, But Typically, You Will Need: *Filled Application Form

Passport-Style Photo

Impressions or Release to Collect previous fingerprints (Background Checks)

* Check for fingerprint release (~$20)*

Photocopy of Birth Certificate or Passport as a proof of citizenship

Application Fee (~$100)

Each state may have various other requirements. Pharmacology requirements are different in each state, but if you have at least one pharmacology class, in most cases, it will suffice. If you haven't taken a specific pharmacology course, you must complete a comprehensive pharmacology form. If you have more than five years since you started the Pharma course, you may have to take the pharmacology course of CEUs and submit it for validation. Some states (like New Jersey) require everyone to use CEU to open controlled substances (New Jersey 6 credits). Again, make sure to read the detailed instructions on the application and strictly follow them.

It will ensure speedy processing without delay. Your State's BON may or may not necessitate you to sign the application from a Notary official. In this case, there will be a Notary Affidavit within the application. Take the document to the courthouse, the UPS Store, or another agency, and get it notarized before submission.

If BON in your state allows applications to be submitted online, fill out the application form as it usually reduces processing time. Alternatively, if your state does not have an online application, you must print the form to send it. Collect all the information you need and send it in a secure envelope. I prefer to send essential documents to BON through the UPS Store, but any service that provides fast service, tracking, and secure delivery is acceptable.

Wait for State Licensure

This stage is always the longest step in the NP certification process. Depending on the effectiveness of your state's BON, this can take a long time. For BON in most states, the average waiting time is said to be 8-12 weeks. However, in some cases, you have to be proactive. If online authentication is available in your state, check online to see if your application is being processed. If eight weeks have elapsed, you must call and receive an update on your application's status.

No matter how long you spend, once you receive a state license, you can apply for DEA and NPI. In many states, you can also apply for a secondary controlled substance permit.

Apply for your DEA License

You can apply for your DEA License through many online portals. It will cost around $731, and the processing time takes 4-6 weeks. You will find an application form on the DEA website. Fill in all the required information, and then pay with a debit or credit card of your choice. Although the license is expensive, it can be used for three years in most states. Besides, you may be able to ask your prospective employer to refund this fee on your behalf.

Apply for your Secondary Controlled Substance License

Many states, including New Jersey, entail a secondary controlled substance license. It is often referred to as Controlled Dangerous Substances (CDS) or Controlled Substances Permits. However, less than half of the states require this license.

You may need to wait for the DEA license to complete before applying for the other license. Your state's BON should also provide this information on its official website. Also, you can search for it online. This licensure cost is usually low (~ $ 20), and the processing time is often 2-4 weeks.

How to Apply for NPI

The National Provider Identifier (**NPI**) is a 10-digit number used to classify you to Medicare and Medicaid Services. To apply for this number, you must fill in the online application form. Create an account, log in, and click 'Apply NPI for myself.' Correctly fill in the information and click submit.

As long as you complete the online application in the approved manner, you will receive your NPI number within ten days, and your request is free. In fact, you can apply for NPI as a nurse, and you can update it once you get the NP license.

Moreover, these are some general problems that you must overcome in the whole NP certification process. After completion, you can formally become a new nurse practitioner to fully exercise your education and training. Each state's situation may be different, so make sure to read the BON website of your state carefully. Some jobs may allow you to work faster. These jobs will make you familiar with the working environment, electronic medical records, and the facility itself. However, you will not be able to see the patient independently until at least your state's consent is obtained.

Tips on Landing the First Job

The first (or second) year of becoming a nurse practitioner may be the most challenging and emotionally exhausting year of your career. You are drawn into a strange environment. Come on, we all know that nursing schools cannot prepare you for the real world of patient care!

You are anticipated to hold the lives of people in your hands right off the bat. This is a challenging task, and it is easy to feel defeated because you are not the perfect graduate specimen.

As a new NP graduate, I experienced a difficult time, especially when my expectations of myself initially met the job's reality. It made me very tired and exhausted. In retrospect, I am proud of my persistence and hard times. Here's what I have learned throughout the process, and what I tell every new NP graduate student experiencing the same thing.

Build Your Support Network Early

In a nursing school, it is easy to teach challenges to our classmates and peers. However, if you do not want to keep in touch with your classmates, teachers, and mentors after graduation, you can easily lose these vital connections. This is why it is so essential to maintain these relationships and build new ones. The support network can provide advice, guidance, and even job opportunities. So, if you haven't already done so, make sure you get the email addresses of all your classmates and teachers. Remember, there is no shame in asking for help. As long as you ask for it, someone could take the opportunity to help you. We've all been there before! Also, if you are not an active member of job posting sites, you should create a profile right away.

Take A Strategic Approach For Your First Job

The first job may not be exactly what you expected, but it's definitely a step in the right direction. You will learn a lot and lay the final foundation for the next few years. Remember, it is easy for NP graduates who do not know professional knowledge to graduate. However, you must understand yourself and should only apply for a job that matches your personality and lifestyle. Don't settle for a job just because you have an offer. The responsibilities of a nurse practitioner are way too important to not be fulfilled in a complete state of awareness. So do not get into jobs that you are well aware you will not be interested in or fill in the gap. For instance, if you know you don't want to work in pediatrics, don't apply in such settings. If you are not good at anything, the float pool is a high starting point. Also, you will have the chance to experience many different majors. If you want to specialize in intensive care units, apply for an ICU job – yes, new graduates will indeed get a professional offer!

Last but not least, connect with your network and build new links. There are several Facebook groups explicitly established for new grad NPs and even for specialties. There are even groups for NPs that wish to be entrepreneurs and start their own practice, infusion clinic, e-commerce site, or brick and mortar store. The support is out there— you just have to look!

Focus On Resume And Cover Letter For Every Job

You should never submit the same old resume and cover letter for every job opportunity. They must be targeted at specific jobs, hospitals, and specialties. Make sure you take the time to distinguish yourself. The final resume guide will help you create the best NP resume and even provide free templates. It will also make clear where exactly you want to see yourself.

Prepare For Your Interviews

Interviews can be nerve-wracking, but they shouldn't be! How? Well, as a fresh NP graduate, preparing for interviews will undoubtedly help. And by prepping, I don't intend you to explore the internet about 'nursing interview questions' and memorize universal responses. There is much more that goes into interview preparation. I can give you some of the questions that you must ask at the time of the interview.

- *How many patients will I see?*
- *What does my training entail?*
- *What is the call schedule?*
- *How does paid time off work?*
- *Do I have to do my own billing and coding?*

What to do before preparing for the interview?

- *Interview question samples and answers to behavioral-based interview questions*
- *Dressing adequately for the interview*
- *Follow up after your interview*
- *Gracefully handle rejection*
- *What to do after you received a job offer*
- *Salary discussions*

Contract Negotiation

Contract or Salary negotiations shouldn't make you uncomfortable. You must remember that as nurse practitioners (NPs), you are a valuable asset to the hiring organization. Speaking of contract negotiations, your knowledge and skills should be in demand.

The contributions of APRNs, NPs, physician assistants, and other senior practice providers help the hospital or clinic make a profit, so you should get fair compensation. New graduates often ask if they should discuss their contracts or not. It is true that the new NPs may have less influence than experienced professionals, but all applicants must negotiate their contract before accepting it.

Consider contract negotiations as a dialogue, not a battle. You are preparing to establish a partnership with a new hospital or clinic. This is your chance to learn the salary structure of the job. Discussions can also give you a clear understanding of how employers will reward your performance monetarily.

Besides, you must understand your pay structure. As nurse practitioners, many of us are paid according to productivity (basically the income we generate from the practice). Such a compensation structure is based on an RVU or relative value unit. Those of us who use the productivity compensation model have a basic understanding of how this system works. At the most basic level, Medicare and other payers reimburse medical providers for the services they provide, based on a specific value assigned to each type of service.

I wish to make you as satisfied with the contract as you are with the new job. Don't settle down for less! If you know what you want, it's important to advocate for yourself from the beginning. Consider the negotiation table as the first step in a productive journey with your new boss.

Treat Yourself Gracefully

Becoming a new NP graduate is like learning to ride a bike. With 13 wheels, drum sets, and crossword bikes, you must complete all operations simultaneously. Be patient with yourself and your mistakes. Treat yourself as a friend, and do not disappoint yourself when you are not as well-informed as someone with ten years of experience. Don't be too hard on yourself; we all learn from experience.

Getting Off Orientation Is Not A Race

If you are employed with other fresh graduates, you will usually look at them and feel like you are competing to be the best new graduate nurse practitioner. Who can care for more patients with higher acuity faster? Who will be put in the post at the earliest? Unfortunately, your work culture can keep this going forever, especially if the manager starts commenting, it will make you feel left out.

Learn to reduce your sensitivity to this situation. If others are progressing, that's fine. If others seem to have more educated patients, so be it. You should emphasize on your journey and fill in the gaps you need. This has nothing to do with winning the game. We all have different speeds and advantages. Believe me; everybody will shine in their time.

It Doesn't Have To Be Your 'Forever Job.'

My first job was in a small family medical clinic and was very fast-paced, and training was nonexistent. I had to refer to my circle of professional friends for advice and what to do in some instances. I did make some mistakes, but they each offered unique learning experiences. I still hold the experiences of that job with me until this day. I took those mistakes home with me, to bed, and to sleep.

You will always ask how I could have done this differently, but understand that you don't have to stay there forever. The clinic had complicated patients and chronic pain patients that other offices did not want to take. The physician on-site had a more liberal approach to controlled medications. His heart was in the right place, and he wanted to please patients. However, it didn't buy him friends in the pharmacy. I personally did not have a DEA license and left the controlled meds for him to manage. Also, I felt like I was tied to the facility forever. I knew that I wanted to explore more, and I wasn't sure what that looked like. Some days are more testing than others. But remember the way your life looks now – specifically if you are having a tough time – doesn't mean it's going to be this way forever. Things are always changing, and individuals come and go in life.

Do Something That Makes You Feel Blissful

When I graduated from the NP's school and began preceptorship, I remember feeling so inadequate and new. I needed something to counterbalance these feelings. So, amid the stress of precepting, I looked for things to relax my mind and divert my attention.

Choose what you like and are good at, whether it's skating, basketball, painting, or gardening. Pick it up again and let it remind you that you can be good at things. Feeling grateful is the key to happiness.

You Are Currently Building Empathy

One day, you will teach someone just like you. Don't let the bitter situation rob you of that experience. Do not let the pain of others continue to spread through you. Remember the feeling right now and tell others what you need now. You must feel empathetic about treating yourself well. Go out, and buy beautiful clothes for yourself. Do anything that makes you feel better.

Big Hospital Systems vs. Private Practice

Most job applicants with an NP's degree know that they want to work in a specific environment. The environment directly impacts on the quality of your work. Different health systems require nurse practitioners to take on various responsibilities, so it is crucial to concede the reasons that differentiate hospitals from private practice. Here are some ways these facilities differ.

Patient Interaction

According to research, one of the most significant differences between private clinics and hospitals is the working relationship between nurse practitioners and patients. Most private facilities are small, and there are fewer licensed doctors than hospitals. Resultantly, the number of patients seen by nurse practitioners in private clinics in a day can be much smaller than in hospitals. Therefore, medical professionals in private practice can often focus on providing high-quality care to a smaller population of patients and understanding them better. The hospitals may require more time. However, it can also allow more freedom of self-management when interacting with patients. Hospitals often require more comprehensive care because patients visit hospitals all the time to assess their health. Private practice generally provides a more relaxed working environment, while hospitals offer more action and alertness.

Nursing Duties

The American Association of Nursing Schools explained that nurse practitioners are the compelling component of hospital staff and the principal care providers in these facilities. Although doctors can diagnose injuries and conditions more often, nurse practitioners are responsible for caring and patient monitoring. Private clinics operate differently, and nurse practitioners provide fewer clinical services than hospitals.

In private clinics, most nurse practitioners' duties are related to updating medical information on electronic health records and other tasks, such as taking blood pressure and performing heart rate measurements. However, in today's era, an NP's responsibilities go beyond these basic operations.

Clinical Experience

Working in a large hospital can be a rewarding and stimulating experience. Nursing degrees indicate that busy schedules and working long hours will cause enormous losses to nurse practitioners. Still, the experience of working in such an organization can have a consequential impact on future opportunities. Caring for various illnesses and injuries can provide nurse practitioners with valuable knowledge and an in-depth understanding of healthcare management. Due to the clinical experience's small scope, private practice often provides greater flexibility. It offers relaxation in shifts and shorter work schedules with paid leave. Fewer patients believe that nurse practitioners can provide personalized attention that is about quality, not quantity.

Work And Home Balance

In my opinion, caring for more patients could be either positive or negative. Sometimes the extra work at the hospital can be exhausting, limiting your energy when spending time with family and friends. The private practice may provide better opportunities to balance your work and social life, schedule management, and reduce workload.

Healthcare can be a profitable industry. Before applying for a vacancy, it is essential to understand the pros and cons of both environments. Consider a shadow nurse in two places to determine the most suitable position for you.

The next imperative thing I want all you readers to ponder is variations in different states. The use of nurse practitioners is a way to address the shortage of primary care providers for doctors. Over the past two decades, the number of NP training and exercise programs has increased. However, the regulations that limit its scope of practice vary from state to state. I would like to assess the impact of state regulations on the increased care provided by NPs in the United States. I found that the number of Medicare patients receiving NP care has increased by 15 times from 1998 to 2010.

By 2010, states with the least restrictive NP practice were 2.5 times more likely to receive NP for primary care than those with the most restrictive NP. Relaxing state restrictions on NP practices should increase their use as the primary care provider. This, in turn, will reduce the national shortage of primary care providers. The full practice authority is the authorization of the Nurse Practitioner (NP). According to the exclusive licensing jurisdiction of the Board of Nursing

(BON), it can evaluate patients. Besides, it allows us to diagnose, prioritize, and interpret diagnostic tests and initiate and manage various treatments. The National education requirements, plan certification, and board certifications are consistent with national standards. To become an NP, you must fulfill these standards. The criteria include a bachelor's degree in nursing, qualifying as a registered nurse (RN), graduating from a nationally recognized NP graduate program, meeting state standards for higher education, and passing the NP Board certification exam. Despite these national standards in nursing, there are still inconsistencies in how state laws and legislative bodies authorize (license) the practice of NPs.

Also, I feel the need to converse from where these variations originated. This variation began in the 1970s when states began to regulate NPs beyond their registered nursing licenses. However, the initial recognition of NP is still essential. Over the past few decades, this patchwork of authorized practice has brought preeminent challenges to the NPs, patients, and healthcare.

The State Practice Environment

As a nurse practitioner, you must clearly understand how the laws and state regulations will affect your practice. The AANP's interactive "state practice environment" map outlines NP licensing in Washington, DC, and 50 states across the United States.

Practice Environment Specifics
Full Practice

First of all, I will expound 'Full Practice.' The National practice and licensing laws allow all NPs to evaluate patients. This evaluation is done under the National Nursing Council's exclusive consent. Full practice will enable NP to examine, command, and interpret analytical tests and authorization to manage the treatment of patients independently from physician oversight. It includes prescription and medication supervision. This is a model recommended by the National Academy of Medical Sciences (formerly known as the Institute of Medicine) and the National Council of Nursing. This allows the NP to practice at their full scope and reduce red tape and barriers to healthcare to patients.

Reduced Practice

In Reduced Practice, the National practice and licensing laws reduce NP's ability to participate in at least one NP practice component. The State law requires an occupationally regulated cooperation agreement with another medical service provider. This will enable the NP to provide patient care. It limits the installation of one or more elements of the NP's practice.

Restricted Practice

Likewise, in Restricted Practice, the National practice and licensing laws limit NP's ability to participate in at least one component of NP practice. Yet, the State law requires another medical service provider to authorize or control the team's career. It restricts an NP's ability to provide independent patient care.

In FPA (Full Practice Authority) states, the NP license does not rely on unnecessary contracts or relationships with doctors or the state medical committee's supervision. As a result, NP (in FPA) is more likely to practice in rural and underprivileged areas. While it meets the highest standards of quality and safety of care, the NP workforce has also increased. Countries that limit or reduce the NP's capacity by limiting licensing agencies are more closely linked to the geographic medical disparities. These disparities include the increased burden of chronic disease, the scarcity of primary care, the rise in medical costs, and the lower position in national health rankings.

This is why the AANP supports the "Consensus Model for Advanced Practice Registered Nurses" and the adoption of the National Nursing Council "Model Practice Act." NPs with FPA must meet the requirements for licensed education. They must maintain national certification and consult and access other healthcare providers when patients need them. NPs must be held accountable to the public and the BON for delivering high standards of care across the country.

FPA States

Nearly half of the US states and territories have passed FPA licensing laws against NP. These include Colorado, Alaska, Arizona, Connecticut, District of Columbia, Guam, Hawaii, Idaho, Iowa, Maine, Maryland, Minnesota, Montana, Nebraska, California, Nevada, New Hampshire,

New Mexico, North Dakota, Northern Mariana Islands, Oregon, Rhode Island, South Dakota, Vermont, Washington, and Wyoming.

How Will It Impact Your Patients And Practice?

Approving FPA for NPs offers patients direct and complete access to all the facilities that they are equipped to provide.

• Improving access opportunities – the FPA has created more access to medical services, especially in cities, rural and underprivileged areas. The states with FPA are more likely to have NP work in rural and the under-supplied regions and NP practices than those with stricter restrictive licensing models.

• Streamline the nursing process and improving nursing efficiency – the FPA provides direct and comprehensive NP services to patients. It eliminates outdated delays of care mainly caused when outdated regulations require an NP as part of an unnecessary statutory mandatory contract.

• Cost reduction – the FPA avoids duplication of service costs and bills due to outdated doctor supervision of the NP practice. It reduces unnecessary duplication of orders, home visits, and nursing services.

- Patient's choice – the FPA allows patients to see the healthcare provider of their choice. It removes anticompetitive licensing restrictions that impede patient-centered healthcare.

The State Dictates The Extent Of Physician Oversight.

Nurse practitioners are professional nurses when it comes to providing care. They have gone through extensive training and medical education. They are equipped to provide a variety of health facilities, like the diagnosis and management of common and complicated medical conditions for people of all ages.

According to statistics from the American Association of Nurse Practitioners, nurse practitioners have provided primary, acute, and specialized medical services to patients of all ages. As of August 2019, there are more than 270,000 licensed practice nurses in the United States. Operational nurses evaluate patients, order and interpret diagnostic tests, diagnose, initiate, and manage treatment plans, including prescribing medicines.

As clinicians, nurse practitioners use clinical experience to diagnose and treat health conditions. They focus on health promotion, disease prevention, and health management. Professionally, executive nurse practitioners express their commitment to providing a comprehensive perspective on healthcare.

Therefore, in this chapter, I would also like to discuss three areas of practice for nurse practitioners: practice authority, prescription authority, and nurse practitioners as primary care providers.

Practice authority can be defined as the ability of nurse practitioners who practice under the supervision or non-supervision of doctors. Some states require the NP to establish relationships with physicians. It outlines the procedures that nurse practitioners can perform, like the duties of consulting doctors. In some states, the policy specifies whether nurse practitioners must complete the transition to practice before starting independent practice. In other states, executive nurse practitioners have completely independent rights of training. It allows them to practice independently without medical supervision.

Prescription authority refers to the jurisdiction of practicing nurse practitioners to prescribe. Some states require physician relationships to outline the nurse practitioner's prescription capabilities. Some states specify whether nurse practitioners must complete the transition to the internship period for independent prescribing. In some places, the state law allows licensed physicians to prescribe medication independently without the need for medical supervision.

Some states unequivocally classify a nurse practitioner as a primary care provider. It can include primary care as a focused objective for a nurse practitioner, whereas some states do not explicitly recognize nurse practitioners as primary care providers.

The Unique CAQH Profile (Council For Affordable Quality Healthcare)

If you have been working in the medical field for some time, you may have heard of CAQH. However, listening to it and really understanding its role are two separate things. Allow me to enlighten you with the unique CAQH profile. There is still a lot of misunderstanding about CAQH, like what it is, what it does, and why it is used. I will answer these questions and tell you the significance of this profile and how to register with it.

Over the years, CAQH has gone through many iterations, but its core services remain the same. They are necessarily a vast database that insurance and certification companies can use for a fee. CAQH will not submit an insurance company application or complete the certification process for you, but they can play a vital role in this process.

Consider your license, Malpractice policy (COI), DEA certificate, or any other content that would typically expire without your intervention. Insurance companies need these files instead of giving every payer an updated license. You can upload this file to CAQH to test its accuracy and provide the payer access to the data. Not all plans can use CAQH, so it's important not to assume that every payer will have your information once a personal profile has been created. It is not available in most local/regional health plans and is not used by government payers. Remember, Tricare, Medicaid, or Medicare do not use CAQH.

When Is CAQH Used?

CAQH is used for payers and initial credentialing. This means it's not a set and forget database, as you need to maintain it yourself. When you first get a health plan certificate, payers sometimes use your CAQH application/configuration file and export it to their system. For this, the payer must be authorized, and they will usually ask for your CAQH ID number by phone, online, or email.

Once you join and start running, including signing a contract (CAQH is not involved in this process), the payer can use CAQH to keep your documents up to date. This makes it vital to remember to re-test every 90 days and update your documentation.

Why You Should Register With CAQH

First of all, many insurance companies need CAQH, so you don't have much choice. There are exceptions because some states have their own systems, and their functions are quite similar to CAQH. However, even if your state has its arrangement (which is rarely true), you can still register with CAQH. Because some counties do not use the state system, and ultimately, they prefer CAQH.

As well as being necessary for most states, it also improves efficiency by reducing the number of unwanted or information requests that have to be processed.

How To Register With CAQH

1. Prepare all documents to upload and update your resume. You will need your license, DEA, and controlled substance certificate (if required), medical malpractice certificate, board certificate, hospital privileges (if applicable), and diploma. You should not start applications if you cannot complete them.

2. Ensure you have three professional references as they are mandatory for your application.

3. If you are starting a practice, the information about your new entity is required. The information includes legal entity information, billing company information if outsourcing tax ID, address (including payment and correspondence if they are different), credentialing contact, billing contact, hours of operation, phone/fax, and group NPI.

4. Once you are confident that you have everything ready for submission, go to the official website to start the procedure.

5. Upon completion of the application, the payer now needs to be given access to the information source. Before they do this, you must submit the signed, verified document provided by CAQH. This is to verify that you have sent the correct information and inform the payer that your claim is ready for review.

6. After announcing/endorsing the signature and date, you must ensure and remember to upload the document.

Make sure you safely keep your CAQH ID, user ID, and password. Remember to check it every ninety days to ensure it does not require any attention. CAQH should email you or anyone you are a credible contact with, but you don't want to rely on their reminders.

Now let's talk about malpractice. I would like to begin with a definition of what malpractice in nursing means. Generally, it is explained as negligence or failure to provide reasonable care to the patient. Nurses Practitioners are often held accountable to this standard. A malpractice suit against an NP claims that the NP did something that caused an injury to a patient.

The National Practitioner Database shows that claims against NPs increased by 18% between 2007 and 2011. The study also shows that the number of allegations leading to serious indemnity has risen by 19% since 2009. The diversity of factors related to an increased likelihood of claims against NPs have enhanced for neglect of duty.

Family NP and adult/gerontologist physician NP have the highest medical malpractice claim rates, while NPs working in an inpatient environment had higher indemnity prices. Compared to states with full prescription authorizations, NPs without prescription authorizations are twice as likely to have a claim against them. Working in an outpatient clinic, treating more than 16 patients a day, and less than six years' experience also increases the likelihood of malpractice claims. The intent is not to worry you, but I want you to be mentally prepared for everything. Besides, it is worth noting that the medical malpractice claims that NPs face are more frequent in states that require physician supervision and administration. According to reports, Florida, California, New York, Massachusetts,

Pennsylvania, Arizona, and Mississippi have a higher rate of NP malpractice claims. Among these areas, only Arizona offers full practice authority to NPs. Caring for patients with more complicated chronic diseases also increases the likelihood of liability claims and medical malpractice.

Since the implementation of the Patient Protection and Affordable Care Act, many NPs are becoming the primary healthcare provider of choice and caring for patients with complex medical problems. They are now working further in more specialized areas, including hospital emergency patients, and taking full responsibility for critically ill patients. All these factors surge our malpractice risk, and this risk drives insurance premium costs up.

However, there is no point in thinking that NPs taking independent accountability for patient care in the upcoming years will increase claims. Lastly, allow me to finish with the NPI number. As previously mentioned, the National Provider Identifier (NPI) will classify health care providers on a state level. This entails that the NPI will be documented by all professionals working in the health care industry. The NPI will swap health care provider identifiers that are currently used. For instance, the NPI will change Medicare legacy numbers, such as UPINs (unique physician [provided] identification numbers) and PINs (personal identification numbers).

The NPI is required because it is a mandatory HIPAA standard, and it simplifies billing. It is a single provider's identification number that will be accepted and recognized by all health plans. Therefore, there is no need to report, maintain, and track multiple providers' identification numbers.

As part of HIPAA, the Health Insurance Portability and Liability Act 1996 contains "administrative simplification" provisions. These regulations set out the requirements for standardized unique identifiers for all medical service providers and health plans covered by HIPAA. CMS (Centers for Medicare & Medicaid Services) developed a system to assign these unique identifiers.

The National Plan and Provider Enumeration System, a part of CMS, offers NPI numbers through the official website. CMS also provides a search service for all NPI records in its free catalog. There are two types of NPI numbers. The first category is for personal service providers, such as doctors, physician assistants, dentists, physiotherapists, and nurses. The second category is suitable for businesses or organizations that provide healthcare services or supplies, such as hospitals, nursing homes, group clinics, laboratories, pharmacies, and home healthcare organizations. Once allotted, the provider's NPI remains with them regardless of location changes or job switches.

How Are NPI Numbers Used?

The NPI numbers are required to obtain reimbursement from insurance companies and prescribe medications. The number is also necessary to refer patients to other health care practitioners that participate in health plans. Summarily, NPI numbers are used by health care providers for:

- *Classifying themselves in HIPAA health care transactions.*

- *Recognizing other health care providers in transactions or correspondence.*

- *Medical prescription.*

The health plan uses the NPI number to communicate with the provider, process the transaction, and coordinate benefits with other plans as needed. An electronic medical records system uses the NPI number to identify treatment providers in medical records. Nurse practitioners have been adequately used in the healthcare system today. Meanwhile, primary care physicians, population growth, and a shortage of elderly patients needing treatment continue to grow their demand. Over the years, the role of nurse practitioners has expanded from routine medical services to sophisticated and professional hospitals and medical practice facilities across the country.

As the NP's role continues to grow and the need to provide quality medical services to a growing population increases, the exposure to risk also elevates. The well-informed public has higher expectations for outcomes, creating an environment that makes it easier for healthcare professionals to take responsibility. With the use of new technologies and electronic medical records, NPs must be more diligent in offering and recording their healthcare services.

Chapter 3
What I Wish I had Known

"Nurses are the heart of healthcare."

–Donna Wilk Cardill

From nursing school to the operating theatre, nurse practitioners are the most respected professionals in healthcare. They stand by a patient's side throughout heart-rending and blissful moments. Every day starts with a new challenge. As a nurse practitioner, I have to encounter many trials during a single working day. Every day, we can witness hundreds of patients, experience birth and death, and make life-altering decisions in seconds.

The job of a nurse practitioner can be appalling when you actually get into it. The vomit, the blood, and the intimidating atmosphere commonly litter the workplace. Still, most nursing students can easily handle these visual horrors. However, many things can come as a surprise when a nursing student gets a job. I was bombarded with loads of new information in the nursing school. I was expected to have it all memorized for the exams a week later.

Many lessons in nursing schools extend beyond the classroom. I wish I could build a time machine and rewind my life. I wish I had known things that would later save me a lot of stress.

The things that I wish I knew before I became a nurse practitioner aren't well-tended secrets. However, they are outcomes of the occupation that you may not comprehend beforehand. That's the reason I want to share some things I experienced as a nurse practitioner. I am confident that my experiences will help you not feel as stressed as I was in my first year.

The job of a nurse practitioner can pretty much look the same after one year. So, it's a matter of the first one or two years. In this chapter, I have compiled some excellent pieces of advice that I wish someone had told me before my nursing journey. Let's begin with some helpful advice to a novice nurse practitioner.

Board Certification

Board certifications are an excellent way to become more confident in your capabilities. These certifications boost your marketability and increase your chances of getting the right job. I highly recommend getting the board certifications as a novice NP. However, the requirements for obtaining these certifications may vary from state to state, with national certification becoming more of the norm. Be certain to find out the procedure for the state where you want to practice. The AANP and the ANCC are the two certifying bodies in the USA. I recommend that you study for three to four months, sit in a review class, and then take the exam soon afterward. Each agency is similarly respected, and it is up to the NP to decide which one they choose. Each of the exams are slightly different in content and questions. Not applying for these certifications creates self-doubt, and fear begins to creep in. Besides, stick to your current job until you sit the exam. Doing this won't make you feel additionally stressed about the new work environment.

Patient Population

"Every Nurse was drawn to nursing because of the desire to care, to serve, or to help."

–Christina Feist Heilmeier

The most essential part of transitioning to the NP role is identifying your first position. Before you start your job hunt, deciding which patient population you would like to serve is imperative. It helps you stay focused and ease your job search. For instance, if you choose to work in a specialty area, such as cardiac, you can quintessence your networking expertise in that area.

Some NPs have been credentialed and practice in the family or adult patient population. Likewise, many choose to practice privileges in hospitals or long-term care facilities. So, my advice is that you decide on your patient population before passing out of nursing school. This way, you will also have much more time to research your ideal patient type.

Contact List

"Networking is more about farming than it is about hunting."

-Ivan Misner

Networking is nothing more than meeting friends. Whether you realize it or not, you're already online every day. When you have a conversation with someone next to you, introduce yourself! Tell people about your profession. Everyone you meet can help you in your job hunt. Get your name in the contact list of other practitioners. Stay in touch with the physicians or NPs with whom you completed your clinical hours. Even if they don't need a new NP when your job search begins, they can still help you with many opportunities. They can recommend your name for many job openings internally. No matter what you do, don't work only to become an NP.

This path can certainly lead to dissatisfaction. Networking can also help others. As human beings, we are keen to establish contact with others. Without these connections, you will become isolated and feel lonely or even depressed. Therefore, the real goal of the network should be to re-energize your existing relationships and develop new ones.

Mining hidden job markets may require more planning and nerves than searching the Internet. Trust me; this is far more effective and useful. Whether in good times or bad moments, networking will help you find the right job. As a novice practitioner, you must establish valuable contacts in your chosen field. It will keep you focused and motivated during the job hunt process.

Job Evaluation

"People need to know how their job contributes."
-W. Edwards Deming

When carefully evaluating potential employers for job interviews, make sure you ask for job expectations. These expectations include patient load, time spent with each patient, and working hours. Additionally, make sure that the services you are required to provide are consistent with the practice of nurse practitioners in your state. Besides, ask about administrative tasks that often include scheduling and paperwork. Moreover, ask for the details of clinical support. It includes assistance with complex patients where you might need help managing.

One study examined the requirements for a successful transition to the NP. It states that the underlying medical practice of adopting new NPs should ensure formal guidance and support from doctors. The senior NPs who are familiar with this role should provide written resources, consultation, and peer support. Ideally, your new work environment should provide all of the required resources. Still, you should ask these questions to stay on track.

Realistic Goals & Expectations

"Expectation is the root of all heartache."

-William Shakespeare

In the transition period, you must never forget that you are only a novice NP. Having impractical expectations of yourself can augment your anxiety about the new role. As mentioned previously, the new NPs suffer from the *"Imposter Phenomenon."*

In this case, you feel that you are not qualified for the job and are duping the boss into believing otherwise. You also feel that your boss will find out one day. To cope up with these feelings, daily reflect on your inner self. At this point, you should identify that the learning curve for a new NP can be steep. You must realize that you are just transitioning from student to RN.

Self-reflection can help you focus on what you're learning, instead of focusing on what you don't know or do wrong. I recommend you to keep a diary for recording your thoughts and problems. Remember, when you become an NP, you play a new professional role.

You are now a primary care provider. Even if you are an experienced senior RN, the role of the PC provider is still new to you. It's normal to question your assumptions and actions in this job. The patient care decisions you make now are different from the past. This can be quite challenging.

Learn from My experience

"Nothing ever becomes real till it is experienced."

-John Keats

To expound the above points, let me walk you through the challenges and barriers I confronted in my first NP role. My first position was in a small family medical clinic where I'd spent some months of my clinical time. On my first day, I had some patients that I found a bit overwhelming. After I voiced my struggle dealing with patients without training, my schedule lightened up a little.

It gave me some time to look up the clinical information I required and finish my charting. I learned through my mistakes. I took them as part of my learning experience. At that time, motivation and consistency kept me going. In some instances, I was much more occupied. However, I continued to raise my concerns regarding the patients' safety. I was cautious whether I could provide thorough care – especially in light of being a new NP. Yet, my schedule didn't allow time to provide adequate care for complex patients. Still, I did what I could to provide the best care under the circumstances.

At times, I didn't get the required guidance as a new NP. Now that I am experienced, I know the answers. The inadequate support caused feelings of insufficiency, job dissatisfaction, and self-doubt. I recognized this wasn't the way I'd envisioned practicing as an NP. Still, I never gave up. Although I continue to feel overwhelmed at times, I know that I must support myself. Some of my training sessions have been incredibly useful, but a specialty requires much on-the-job learning and independent reading.

Time Value

"The two most powerful warriors are patience and time."

-Leo Tolstoy

Even in the best case, the transition to NP can be tough. The best advice I can offer is to recognize that it takes time to adjust to the new role. Give yourself some time to ease your anxiety and self-doubt. Setting realistic goals, letting employers have realistic expectations for you, and having strong peer support can also make this transition smooth. To solve the problem of unrealistic expectations in a broader scope, we must educate the medical community about the role of the NP.

We should emphasize that we are not doctors, and we cannot expect ourselves to practice as one. NP and physician roles have some similarities, but there are marked differences, too. Find a collaborating physician willing to spend time to understand what an NP is and what to do and be patient during the transition. These are the secrets to your success as a solo practitioner.

Insurance Companies' Red Tape

Insurance companies create unnecessary burdens and red tape. As NPs, it makes our jobs much more challenging. Besides, we have to put in the proper ICD-10 code. It contains codes for signs, symptoms, diseases, abnormal findings, social circumstances, complaints, and external causes of injury or disease. The excessive details and different procedures of every hospital make it even more frustrating. The Payers' prior-authorization (PA) requirements delay t? he patient's treatment. It negatively affects clinical outcomes and can lead patients to abandon treatment. Health plan cost-control process, and prior authorization, restricts access to drug treatments and other clinical services. This process requires nurse practitioners to obtain approval before delivering the prescribed medication or ordered service to qualify for payment.

Make the most of your experience

"Personal experience is the basis of all real literature."

– George Henry Lewis

Your clinical experience is really your goal. This point cannot be sufficiently emphasized. Write a rare diagnosis, abnormal lab work, or vague physical examination findings, and study them whenever possible. Also, try to take benefit of these findings. Practice presenting a brief history and physical exam results to your presenter.

Most importantly, practice your own treatment and differential plans. Do not allow your work to merely be a shadow experience. Test yourself by seeing complicated and annoying patients. Note the details and ask questions about anything you don't understand. As a new NP, you must make the clinical experience a valuable part of your education.

Self-Care

"Self-Care is not selfish. You cannot serve from an empty vessel."

–Eleanor Brown

You've heard about it in nursing school, and it's no different in hospital. Taking care of yourself and removing all obstacles is essential to your happiness. Set aside at least a day and a half or even a night each week to turn off your laptop and books. Do something interesting, and in short, forget about all your worries.

For those who like sports, I encourage you to take some time to stay active. In graduate school, especially when studying medicine, it's easy to feel overwhelmed. Look for healthy ways to reduce the pressure in school. One way is to re-establish contact with friends or loved ones. It will sustain your life for a long time.

Things I Wish I Had Known

Hopping onto something new is always scary when you don't have all the facts. That's precisely why choosing a nursing career is so perplexing. It doesn't mean that you can just spend a few years in nursing school and try out a job.

After becoming a nurse practitioner, you can't simply switch your profession. Well, at least not without adequate training and education! Being a registered nurse (RN) is no different. We believe we know the role of RN based on TV shows or our actual interactions with them in hospitals or doctors' offices. But what happens behind the scenes? Once you're on the other side, is the nursing school worth it?

What does it feel like to be a nurse practitioner? It is not easy to understand this profession clearly without talking to those who walk in it. So, to help, I have gathered some facts I wish I had known earlier.

It Can Be Hard On Your Family

Perhaps, your family is very supportive of your desire to be a nurse practitioner, but it can be hard on them. Many nurse practitioners and family members do not know that having a nurse at home can cause stress. NPs work weekends, holidays, and evenings when others are resting. While some nurse practitioners work 12 hours per shift, taking a vacation, or trying to adjust to family time between naps can take up to four days off. Because of the pressure of providing care, some relationships can break. Your emotions may be affected, which will disturb your family. Many nurse practitioners may not see their children when they want because of their work schedules. The only solution to this problem is by actively managing your time. Still, it will be tough for your family members.

How Easily People Forget

The sacrificing attitude is one of the greatest benefits of the nursing profession, but it can also be excruciating. Most people don't appreciate that nurse practitioners sacrifice their eating and avoid going to the bathroom, only to take care of a small need of their patient. People easily forget the kindness you offer them. This can be so agonizing that NPs sometimes turn to the point of harming their own health. Although I put emphasis on the importance of passion in nursing, the pain in it is real. I certainly experienced this pain and wanted to quit nursing altogether. Perspectives on how caring can affect your passion or goals will help you persevere in challenging times. This way, you can develop a good nursing self-care practices to ensure that you do not sacrifice your health.

Bullying Environment

In the nursing world, it is very common to find older, more established nurse practitioners treating new employees poorly. I surely hope it doesn't happen to you. Still, I advise you to be mentally prepared for this case. There are some ways you can learn to prevent being a target.

Make sure you understand your rights as a professional and do not tolerate abuse in the workplace. Naturally, some nurse practitioners want to make a good impression, but some behaviors are never good.

As a new NP, you need support from the more experienced nurse practitioners. So, I can't encourage you to ruin your relationship with them. That doesn't mean you should endure bad behavior at work. All I am saying is to be mentally prepared and wisely make your decisions.

You Can Find Dayshifts

A common belief in the medical profession is that everyone must spend time on night shifts in their job. But that's not true! However, the specific employment situation will vary from region to region. Still, there are no rules prohibiting new NPs from finding a job in dayshifts.

Many local hospitals also accept new graduates for specialized and intensive care jobs. That I used to think was not common practice.

No One Cares How You Feel

This was quite challenging for me to understand. Trying to speak with friends and family is almost impossible. No one really understands what nurse practitioners experience or how we feel. No one realizes what we are going through. Despite this frustration, the fact that you find a friend who really appreciates your experience in nursing school is also encouraging. Finding this support system is everything.

You Have To Remember Everything

You have to remember everything, including the memorizing of your patients' room numbers, names, and medical details. As a nurse practitioner, you must be responsive to their lab results, medications, and vital signs. The doctors can examine patients anytime; make sure you are prepared, as well. If you believe you can't trust your memory all the time, you should keep a notebook. That way, you remember everything about your patient.

Social Life

As a nurse practitioner, your social life is dead. The extended working hours and critical jobs do have an impact on social life. It is indeed essential to balance your social and professional life. The nursing profession demands the best out of you. It leaves you tired and takes up your whole day. Besides, you can't say "No" to any patient as it is unethical. Simply put, this profession leaves your social life in a mess. This can especially happen if you are not prepared in advance.

Extreme Pressure

The one thing that sincerely stunned me about life as a nurse practitioner was how well I worked under pressure. It is not an easy profession – it requires both mental and physical stamina to make it through extended shifts. But if you are passionate, you can make an impact on a patient's life. If you are not up for the job, it's easy to feel burdened. You will be under severe stress concerning the tasks you must finish during your shift.

It's Fine To Make Mistakes

It's alright that you don't know everything. Learning in nursing school for years doesn't offer complete assurance that you're thoroughly prepared for the job. Even senior nurse practitioners still come across medications and cases that are new to their ears. Make it a habit of asking if you have doubts. Confessing that you don't know everything doesn't make you any less of an NP. On the contrary, it makes you better!

The Busy Shifts

Nurse practitioners have so many different errands and tasks that they are recurrently prioritizing. It is one of the most demanding professions, but the rewards are inexpressible. Despite all this, the job comes with a hectic schedule. However, experienced NPs can effortlessly manage their time. As a novice, you must adopt certain habits to manage your busy shifts.

I hope my words have presented some new insight or notions on how to survive and make the best of your NP program. I wish you the best of luck in your studies and the start of your new career. Don't forget that our profession requires consistent learning. Never hesitate to question yourself, check clinical guidelines or clinical references, or consult fellow practitioners when you are not certain.

Chapter 4
How COVID-19 Has Impacted the Profession

"After all, it really is all of humanity that is under threat during a pandemic."

-Margaret Chan

The pandemic is not merely a severe public health problem. It has also triggered catastrophic socio-economic and political crises all over the world. Besides, being the greatest threat to global public health in this century, COVID-19 is also considered a pointer of inequality and the lack of social development.

Let me begin by telling you where and how this pandemic was originated. The first COVID-19 case was reported in Wuhan, Hubei Province, China, in December 2019. Most of the initial outbreaks were related to point-source infections in the wholesale seafood market. Since then, the disease has quickly swept the world and eventually affected every continent except Antarctica. The World Health Organization (WHO) categorizes it as a pandemic (WHO, 2020). The

International Committee for Viral Taxonomy (ICTV) named coronavirus severe acute respiratory syndrome virus 2 (SARS-CoV-2). COVID-19 belongs to a large, diverse family of viruses. It can be classified into four genera, namely, α-, β-, γ-, and δ. The viruses of this family are responsible for the worldwide spread of many pandemics, namely MERS-CoV, SARS, and SARS-CoV-2 that are β-coronaviruses. The global outbreaks of COVID-19 caused a large number of morbidities and fatalities. It also incurred a financial loss of billions of dollars.

If I compare it to the previous diseases and their respective burdens, COVID-19 has caused much suffering than any other infectious disease in the whole world.

In this chapter, I will highlight the impact of COVID-19 on society, and especially on the nursing profession.

COVID-19 Vs. Health

The link between our health and disease is not a new topic. The emergence of COVID-19 in China has caused a substantial global outbreak. It is a massive public health problem with global implications. The virus is highly transmissible and can spread through droplets and close contact. Person-to-person spread of a virus occurs due to close contact with infected people. That's why we must maintain a safe distance from other people having symptoms. These symptoms include dry cough, fever, sore throat, chest pain, and shortness of breath.

COVID-19 Vs. Economy

The loss of precious lives due to the virus causes irrevocable damage to society. On top of this, COVID-19 has harshly demobilized the global economy. Many affected countries have decided to take the necessary measures to limit the spread of the virus. In different countries, major international flights and all forms of business transport have been suspended.

Due to the lockdown, all domestic flights, rail services (excluding food trucks), and all sorts of transport stopped. However, special exemptions are given for those items associated with basic necessities. In almost every country hit by COVID-19, educational, commercial, spiritual, and sports institutions are closed. Except for industries related to basic amenities, all other sectors have suffered a lot. People in the tourism and transport industries face the greatest challenges. Their business level has gone below zero. The economy of many giant countries is now facing the threat of high inflation and rising unemployment. The saddest part is that we cannot blame anyone for this. I am well aware of the fact that many companies are downsizing their employees. However, it is understandable because they have minimum revenue, with the production level below an acceptable level. In this pandemic, the employer has no other option but to downsize its workforce.

The lockdowns are not a favorable option for any country's economy.

It will unswervingly affect the GDP of every nation. Each month, annual GDP growth loses about 2%. The tourism sector alone is facing a decline in productivity of up to 50% to 70%. According to the World Trade Organization (WTO) and the Organization for Economic Co-operation and Development (OECD), the COVID-19 virus is the biggest threat to the global economy.

Some experts say that human civilization has not confronted such a record-breaking disaster after World War II. So, COVID-19 has unquestionably set forth a remarkably terrible influence on the everyday life of humans and the world's economy.

The Environmental Effect

From the beginning, we have manipulated nature for our own benefit. To satisfy the increasing demand of the population, urbanization became unavoidable. The outcome of urbanization hence proved to be detrimental to the global environment. To derive the nature of our whims and desire, we have destroyed nature in many ways.

"We won't have a society if we destroy the environment."

-Margaret Mead

The unavoidable outcome of environmental pollution has become a significant issue of the present day. However, because of the unusual occurrence of COVID-19, almost every country is under partial or total lockdown. Literally, every local administration agency around the world prohibits citizens from leaving their hometown. They are stopping people from avoiding the communal spread of the virus. Various industries are not operating, and all sorts of traveling are prohibited. We all have witnessed that restricting the unnecessary movement has a positive impact on the global environment. The pollution levels of tourist attractions, such as forests, beaches, and hilly areas, have also dropped considerably. The ozone layer has improved to some extent. The pandemic showed diametrically opposite results for human civilization. In a sense, the pandemic caused global devastation, but on the other, it showed a positive impact on the world's environment.

Environmental change is one of the most significant and vital challenges of the 21st Century. In spite of all our efforts to restore nature, we could move a few steps forward. However, during the last few months, the pandemic's consequences have successfully helped the environment to a large extent.

Whatever the cause or the origin, the emergence of COVID-19 emphasizes the positive connection between humans and nature. We must control the source of the disease, cut off the transmission pathway, and use existing drugs and methods to manage the disease's progression. Like all previous disasters on earth, I want to keep everyone optimistic that human beings will definitely defeat this epidemic at the right time.

The Impact On The Nursing Profession

The COVID-19 pandemic has affected the physical and mental health of medical personnel. Specifically, nurse practitioners are more susceptible to COVID-19 infection than the general population due to frequent contact with affected individuals. They are required to work under pressure. There is a lack of proper protective equipment, and NPs must make difficult ethics-related decisions.

In recent months, the world has begun to recognize and acknowledge that nurses are true warriors of the society. However, despite all the praise and honor from our healthcare providers, these are merely words for thousands of nurse practitioners. Remember, bare words buy no barley!

The fact that nurse practitioners are jeopardizing their lives every day to fight coronavirus isn't gaining much attention. Only a few people can tell that nurse practitioners aren't just asked to sacrifice their mental and physical health. They are being asked to sacrifice economically in the face of the pandemic as well. Hence, this chapter also discusses the profound economic impact of the COVID-19 pandemic on nurses, specifically, NPs. It also provides strategies for minority nurse practitioners to guard themselves physically and financially during this pandemic and beyond.

Expendable

Nurse practitioners worldwide, especially in the United States, are required to risk their lives and health. They must work and care for infected patients without the most basic protective equipment. At the same time, they are facing job layoffs along with other problems.

However, NPs not called to the frontlines are facing job losses. The minority nurse practitioners are contending with increasing rates of infection. These NPs put their lives in danger and are targets who can spread the virus in their own communities. This conforms to minority nurse practitioners who may have been exposed to the virus are now facing the prospect of illness. Additionally, they deal with colossal expenses of treatment on a reduced income and possibly without health insurance.

Intensified Risk

We risk our lives to save yours!

Today, nurse practitioners are facing a loss of income and insurance. The coronavirus pandemic has also fundamentally changed the way healthcare is delivered, which increases the physical and financial risks that NPs must face.

For instance, as the virus began to spread, and lockdowns became more fruitful nationwide, healthcare providers progressively turned to telehealth. They found it the best way to show care for their patients. They believe that it has great benefits in ensuring continuity of care while preventing the spread of the virus.

However, telehealth is a new beast for many nurse practitioners. It puts them in more responsibility than they face in the clinics. Perhaps the new technology is effective, but it cannot simulate the conditions of face-to-face patient checks. Many things can be overlooked when using technology. You can't touch the patient, observe how they are walking into the room, or listen to their breathing, so there is a heightened chance of mistake.

My point is not about making mistakes or failing to recognize symptoms. The question is, how many of these mistakes will be judged as malicious and who will take on the financial and legal responsibility. This is of particular concern to nurse practitioners caring for patients with substance abuse disorders. The lockdown has imposed that such patients in recovery transition to telehealth. However, it is well known that drug abuse diseases tend to relapse. The signs of relapse are often challenging to detect, primarily through remote care. If a patient is taking an overdose over auspices of telehealth, the NP could be made responsible for this mistake. So, we all have to be quite cautious about telehealth.

Planning To Switch

It doesn't matter how much loss this pandemic brings to your physical, emotional, and financial situation, there is hope. However, if someone is jobless due to a pandemic, they might think of changing the profession. They simply cannot tolerate the conditions required to endure. Such nurse practitioners are inclined to change their careers.

They don't have to leave the nursing profession entirely. If they still believe that nursing is their passion, they should take the hard lessons and use them for good. There is a possibility that finding a new job would require problem-solving. It might break a person emotionally. Finally, nurse practitioners are being acknowledged as true warriors.

Still, it doesn't make their work any easier. They should enjoy even greater attention as they are at the forefront of the healthcare industry. On the contrary, NPs are experiencing job layoffs, hazardous working conditions, and other financial burdens. Most nurse practitioners are readjusting themselves in a new situation.

As a nurse practitioner, I can't help but wonder how the consequences of the current COVID-19 crisis are affecting the nursing industry as a whole. I envisage the situation after COVID-19 as having one of two opposing trajectories, a rise in the current nursing shortage, or a major influx into nursing.

Sadly, I am scared of the deficiency. The COVID-19 crises might endanger the nursing profession. It can cause a shortage that no country has ever seen.

Who in the right state of mind would want to become a nurse practitioner after this pandemic?

To me, this seems a reasonable question to ask. However, it is essential to identify there is no trial version of nursing. It is simply not possible to put one nursing facility into another and expect the same result. All nurse practitioners might know how to prevent the virus. Yet not every nurse practitioner is prepared to give an IV to an infected individual. I also believe that media should play a significant role in identifying the various skills they need from NPs. Doing this can make nurses more courageous and confident. I understand that it is challenging to convey such good moods during crises. Perhaps, my point merely acts as anticipatory guidance for future management of such pandemics.

What should the public do to help nurse practitioners who are battling this pandemic?

The public can support nurse practitioners in two primary ways. NPs and all healthcare professionals have experienced a severe shortage of personal protective equipment in providing important care to frontline COVID-19 patients. The public can contact local, state, and federal officials to do everything possible to increase the distribution of PPE, thereby highlighting the serious deficiency that medical staff is facing.

Second, the public should stay at home. Even in areas where there is no obligation to stay at home, the public must follow the recommendations. Restricting social interaction is the cheapest way to slow the spread of the virus and make it easier for nurse practitioners and other health professionals on duty.

The Pros & Cons Of The Pandemic

"I have always tried to turn every disaster into an opportunity."

-John D. Rockefeller

The virus has brought the world to a grinding halt. People have lost their loved ones. The pandemic has left many to trails of tears and uncertainty. Despite all this, I continue to walk with positive resilience and realistic optimism.

There is always an opportunity in every disaster. Similarly, there are some advantages and disadvantages of this virus. It will certainly change the world by its end. The good side of this pandemic is that it has made people more aware of their hygiene. They have started self-caring to avoid the COVID-19. Everyone is practicing social distancing and spending time with their families. So, let's move on to the pros and cons of this virus.

Pros
Creativity

"Everything you can imagine is real."

-Pablo Picasso

I believe one of the benefits is increased creativity. The first thing to note is that not everyone can enjoy this benefit. From doctors to brave workers in the supply chain, the available free time is quite variable. People at risk (or unemployed) focus on more urgent needs. However, many people who work from home, who don't commute or meet face-to-face, have more time on their hands. Some families are engaged in different activities. Some of them are quite enjoyable, like board games, puzzles, and jigsaws.

Self-Discipline

With self-discipline, everything is possible. All it takes is a strong will, not only for yourself but for the country as well. At the critical time of COVID-19, the key factor is how people respond to the crisis. They can slow its impact. The World Health Organization (WHO) distinguishes the value of human behavior in controlling epidemics. From the people to the government, the responsibility for self-discipline should be publicized at all levels. In this unprecedented challenge, countries, partners, governments, and systems must provide social and economic protection to vulnerable and marginalized individuals.

Family Time

Most people are working remotely from home and have children as well. So, how can you prevent them from saying, "I'm bored?"

Obviously, I want everyone to continue watching T.V., but not all day. If you're at home, you can make the most of it by spending quality time with your family. Schedule a family dinner. Bake some cookies and bread. There are numerous options available. I don't want you to implode by having too many of them, but you should do anything that makes you happy.

Telemedicine

Covid-19 gives us no choice but to distance ourselves from society. This opens up a new way for us to continue to provide patient care through virtual medicine. The highlights of telemedicine are increasing efficiency, convenience, and reducing exposure to COVID-19. The art of taking a detailed medical history to form a judgment has been refreshed. The relaxation of government policies for billing has helped in ensuring patient care while practicing at the same time.

Improved Expertise

With limited PPE and resources, we have improved our expertise. The doctors and nurse practitioners have become experts at reorganizing resources. We have categorized them as urgent, elective, and emergent. We have taken a step forward to question if a diagnostic test is really required or not. I hope to continue using the same approach in the U.S even after the pandemic. I want the health care system "Need-Driven" rather than "Revenue Driven."

Gentleness

Global suffering has led us to become kind to others. The pandemic has encouraged us to build bridges across geographical barriers. We are more sensitive to other's difficulties because we are all on the same boat. Setting up a support program to discuss post-traumatic stress disorder and stress, wearing masks, and volunteering to provide help are just some of the gestures that arise from this common pain.

Temporary Expansions

Many countries are suffering from nurses' shortages in the middle of COVID-19. According to the reports, the world needs approximately six million nurses to achieve global health targets. To combat the pandemic, many states in America are fast-tracking full practice for nurse practitioners. The states are waiving or suspending collaborative practice agreement requirements for NPs. As a result, temporary expansions are given for serving nurses to meet the current shortfall.

Humility

The philosophical aspect of life is the foundation. Humans are not invincible, and life is unpredictable. The pandemic allows us to understand these distant states clearly. We understand that nature should not be taken for granted.

Nobody would have predicted this virus six months ago. No one had an idea of how this virus will affect our lives. Being modest keeps us on our guard without leading a careless life.

Financial

Being in control of your expenses is a great stress reliever.

We have learned the value of careful handling of finances and savings under economic pressure. "Saving money for rainy days" is a timely proverb in these times. At the same time, people's hearts have also opened to pursue philanthropy.

Advocacy

Demographics highlight the racial and economic differences in COVID-19's survival and outcomes. It shows us another reason for pursuing equality. Sometimes, healthcare policies do not seem to reflect doctors' scientific views adequately. The pandemic shows again that doctors must be more involved in healthcare policies, rather than staying silent.

Renewed Respect

During these turbulent times, the world has recognized the selfless service of medical staff. While we do not want to win awards, gratitude has inspired a spirit of service. Now, people have realized that nursing is not an easy job. It's a job that requires you to put your life in danger.

Cons

The virus has put millions of people on edge. Everybody, including me, was unexpectedly placed in a state of emergency. I assumed I was prepared. My family is healthy, sheltered at home, and good. Having experienced a volcanic eruption, massive earthquake, hurricanes, and typhoons, we thought this would not be as ruthless. Time slowly shifted from one week to another. After a month or two, my optimism slowly began to fade away. It became harder for everyone to stay positive. I started to think more about the cons of the COVID-19 virus.

Confusion

The parents were not adequately prepared. When the schools suddenly closed, most parents were at a loss and ill-prepared. They have no option but to homeschool their children. For students, teachers, and parents, it has always been a steep learning curve in managing 'Virtual Learning.' There is still a state of confusion about schools. However, many schools are considering reopening, but nothing has been concretized. The medical personnel around the world turned to each other on fighting a novel virus. What is the best medication? How to control spread? The most susceptible population? Generally, such questions were answered by random meta-analyses. But on the brink of an illness, we now have a disease with no known treatment.

Currently, all treatments are trial based. The CDC still publishes recommendations almost every other day. It is a challenge for all of us. Are we skilled enough to function in uncertainty? Not being able to provide any authentic medicine is quite distressing.

Double Shifts For Women

In most families, women are in charge of the household. They bear most of the responsibility of keeping the house in order. Never has it been more prolonged than during this pandemic! It is the same in nursing families. They take on the heavy responsibility of family work along with professional responsibilities. In addition to the logistics of handling daily family education and grocery shopping, they must now handle increasing issues.

Lack Of Support

The schools and daycares are closed. Still, most health care workers are expected to report to work. Grandparents who smoothed the babysitting were suddenly out of the picture as we try to limit their social exposure. The baby sitters are reluctant to come out due to fear of contact. Many are stuck between homeschooling/childcare and clinical schedules.

Fear and Anxiety

The biggest fear of most medical staff is taking the coronavirus home. I started wearing scrubs and began a new ritual. I had to remove my clothes in the laundry room and then went directly to the shower room for complete "decontamination." This ensures that I take all possible preventative measures to avoid infection or exposure to family members.

Shortages

The media has compared the medical community's fight with pandemic to war metaphors. In light of the PPE shortage, we are like soldiers without guns. The testing kits were not available. Even the nurse practitioners or healthcare professionals who were uncovered could not get tested. Every hospital gradually realized how ill-prepared they were with the unavailability of beds, staff, and ventilators.

Triage

In many states, hospitals were instructed to stop elective procedures. They were mandated to stop clinical visits during the initial weeks. Finding a balance between risk and benefit had become stressful. With such a confused state of mind, the medical staff was required to perform their duties continually.

Lack of Academic Productivity

In the pandemic, the lack of academic productivity was observed. Research says that women are already not academically as productive as our men. The research productivity of women has taken a backseat in this pandemic. The reason is women are handling both clinical work and maintaining the household.

Financial

The pandemic also caused a rapid economic collapse. The hospitals are not immune to the financial downturn. Many optional treatments and clinical visits were stopped in the pandemic. As a result, doctors and other medical staff experienced pay reductions.

Anger

Conspiracy theorists started screaming, *"It's all fake!"* Such coronavirus deniers believe the epidemic is a scam and completely ignored social distancing. They continue to spread misinformation, causing problems for the rest of the population. It caused anger in many healthcare workers who are sacrificing their lives and their families.

Isolation

"Man is, by nature, is a social animal."

Social distancing further goes on to produce social isolation. I must say I miss my friends. I miss eating out and traveling to different places. This obligatory, but still scarce, new reality has affected many people. It has triggered PTSD, fear, substance abuse, anxiety, and loneliness.

Sadness and Disappointment

This pandemic requires a coordinated approach across the country (even if not globally). Because of all the uncertainty and the lack of direction, necessary leadership skills are more in demand. The lack of coordination has led to increased deaths and the inability to *"flatten the curve."*

Seeing how fragile deadly viruses can control the world, it will never be the same. It won't be the same, even after this evil enemy has retreated. The deaths, loss of income, economic recession, global turmoil, and an uncertain future make us sad.

However, hope is a powerful tool, especially in these hard times. Today, the world is experiencing the COVID-19 crisis, a pandemic that has changed the lives of millions of people. In such critical times, only hope can be an influential source of reassurance. Many people are locked at home, while some are working to help and prevent the virus. Also, everyone needs comfort and the hope that:

We shall overcome this.

Chapter 5
Where is the Profession Going?

"If you don't change direction, you may end up where you are heading."

-Lao Tzu

Fortunately, the nursing industry is heading in the right direction despite the fluctuating trends. It is one of the most in-demand and exciting jobs in America today. Medical professionals work to prevent disease, promote health, and help patients fight illnesses.

The profession advocates health education for patients, families, and communities. When offering direct patient care, nurse practitioners observe, evaluate, and record patient symptoms, reactions, and improvements. They collaborate with physicians to provide the best treatment available. Medical professionals continually seek ways to provide the best possible care for patients. Another crucial element is that doctors and nurse practitioners must relentlessly learn technological advancements to ensure they offer the best patient care. The nursing industry is evolving with new methods and digital innovations. I must say, as a nurse practitioner, you should maintain pace with these changes. You must also ensure that your patient care is up to the mark with this evolution. The responsibility lies on our shoulders. So far, in my experience, I have observed some changing trends. I believe understanding these trends will make the job easier.

First of all, I will discuss the *Shifting Demographics*. Historically, nursing demographics in the United States have been relatively uniform in terms of race and gender. However, the composition of the industry is changing. As per the research conducted in 1930, only 2% of nurses were male. As of 2015, the ratio between men and women was around 9.5:1.

This trend of diversification is also evident in the racial makeover of the industry. Besides, one report was published in 2015 by Dr. Peter McMenamin – an economist at the American Nurses Association. The study found that 77% of registered nurses over the age of 70 were white. Still, among nurses under 40, about 65% were identified as white. In the future, this trend may continue to affect the nursing industry.

The second trend is improved *Leadership Opportunities*. It includes the availability of higher positions regarding better academic qualifications. As per the labor statistics, the demand for nurse anesthesiologists, midwives, and nurse practitioners is expected to increase by 31%. It will probably increase the job market by around 53,400 new jobs.

This trend is coherent with the goals set forth by the Institute of Medicine for nursing. Nursing professionals build a culture of health within communities. So, it is exceptionally vital to support them in leadership roles. As a nurse, we know how to keep people healthy. We want everybody to have a deep appreciation of our value and importance in all health care settings.

Thirdly, I would like to expound on the growing role of *Informatics*. As technology advances, the amount of healthcare data collected through information technology also increases. Some examples include electronic health records, patient portals, and data from wearable devices. The information is then analyzed and used to make appropriate changes to existing clinical procedures and strategies. This trend has a significant impact on a hospital's nursing practice and other U.S. nursing facilities. An increasingly important role of informatics is to change the way nurse practitioners record and communicate information to patients. It also ensures coordinated care and develops evidence-based practice. The growing popularity of informatics has also created a space for professionals. There are job vacancies for people who want to focus solely on the intersection of nursing and data. Some specific jobs held by nursing professionals include:

- *Nursing informatics analyst*
- *Nursing informatics specialist*
- *Clinical analyst*
- *Clinical informatics specialist*
- *Clinical informatics coordinator*
- *Clinical informatics manager*

As health information technology continues to gain popularity, nurse practitioners will be more likely to become involved. Then comes the emphasis on *Population Health*. It is an extensive method of health care. It focuses on the health of the entire population. Although strategies vary by environment, the concept remains the same in this field. It comprises community-wide initiatives. It typically consists of educating primary school students on the importance of maintaining a healthy diet. It also includes encouraging older people in the city to get flu vaccines and other health measures.

As per (HRSA), some outcomes of population health include:

- *More physical activity*
- *Fewer workdays lost to illness.*
- *Less infant mortality and preterm births*
- *Fewer cases of diabetes*

These strategies not only improve health but also save patients' money. The saved resources can be used to prevent medical problems before more expensive interventions are needed. The HRSA states that nurses can bring substantial value to this model of healthcare through the specialized care they provide.

The specialist care they provide can help the system to meet the needs of individuals and groups of patients. The nurse practitioners are well-placed. They can identify problems that need to be addressed extensively. Also, it will connect patients to specific services provided by the community.

The sixth trend is the *Changed Setting*. The hospitals are considered as the most traditional workplaces for nurse practitioners. However, the new truth is that nurse practitioners can now work in a variety of places and settings. They can work in outpatient service centers, specialist clinics, and private centers. As healthcare evolves, so does the environment for hiring nursing professionals.

Today, nurse practitioners work with patients online. With the help of telemedicine technology, nurse practitioners and other healthcare providers can provide virtual advice. They can speak to patients who cannot make appointments in person. With the increasing popularity of this technology, more NPs are finding remote consulting in their list of duties.

The Future Implications

The *Future of Nursing* discusses the roles, responsibilities, and education of nurse practitioners. This part expounds on what NPs should do to meet the growing demand for their services. So, I have compiled some implications that you may see in the upcoming years.

Online Programs Will Gain Popularity.

In 2010, IOM selected the Committee on the Future of Nursing to fabricate future recommendations. They came up with them as action-oriented responses to some of the challenges faced by the nursing industry. One of the propositions was to increase education. The advice focused on improving the percentage of workers possessing a BSN degree from 50 to 80% by 2020.

Considering these changes, the motivation for nurse practitioners to obtain higher education becomes stronger than ever. Online degree programs provide a feasible way to learn. In these programs, NPs can focus on training while continuing to work full time. With this implication, nurse practitioners don't have to sacrifice work-related responsibilities or family obligations to realize higher education. I expect the online MSN-FNP and the post-master FNP certificate programs to increase in the upcoming years.

The Demand Will Increase

One research states that the United States could face a shortage of nurses. In 2032, the study expected a shortfall of up to 56,000 primary care physicians. The reason for this shortage is the aging population. I certainly believe, without enough healthcare workforce, the demand will increase, specifically in the FPA states. In 2018, the AANP stated that the numbers of NPs have reached up to 248,000. I am sure these numbers will continue to rise.

States Will Grant NPs Full Practice Authority

In response to the shortage, more states will permit NPs to practice full authority. At present, 22 states, including Washington, D.C., allow them to work independently. However, other states need an agreement with senior physicians and have restrictions.

Considering the demand, the National Academy of Medicine and the National Council of State Boards of Nursing approve that states must provide FPA. After their approval, the remaining states have no proper reason to restrict authority. So, I predict that states will grant FPA to NPs.

Nursing Jobs Will Grow

Save one life; you're a hero. Save a hundred lives; you're a nurse.

The numbers speak for themselves. All around the world, especially in our country, the shortage is expected to intensify. The older generation needs more care as time passes. With this demand, there will be countless job openings for nurse practitioners. That's Good News!

As per the Bureau of Labor Statistics, RN is one of the best occupations for job growth by 2028. The job openings are estimated to grow by 12%. The BLS mentions 371,500 new RN jobs will be added by the year 2028. Considering these projections, I am hoping for a good outlook for registered nurses in the upcoming years.

Salaries Will Rise

According to one survey in 2018, nurses appear to be benefiting with the increased demand. Around 60% of respondents confirmed that their salaries have been raised in the last few months.

Economic principles state the relationship between demand and earning. As the demand for nurses grows, so should the earnings. It's no surprise that U.S. News ranked RN and NP as 19th and 7th in the "100 Best Jobs" of 2019. Amidst the pandemic, the demand will undoubtedly grow.

Naturally, I expect additional salary raise for NPs in the upcoming years.

Higher Education Will Become The Norm

I expect to see growth in the number of nurses pursuing higher education. Many independent studies show that an increase in the RNs holding at least a BSN degree drops the risk of patient death. More education leads to better outcomes. So, I expect higher education nursing degrees to become the norm for RNs in the upcoming years.

More States Will Join ENLC

The ENLC – Enhanced Nurse Licensure Compact was first implemented in January 2018. It was coordinated with the National Council of State Boards of Nursing (NSCBN). It makes it easier for traveling nurses to work in different states.

The latest state to sign the compact is Indiana. Many states, including Alabama, Michigan, Massachusetts, Vermont, New York, New Jersey, and Rhode Island will join the list quite soon. So, I expect a couple of more states to join the ENLC in the upcoming years.

Telehealth Will Increase

"Innovation is the ability to see change as an opportunity—not a threat."

-Steve Jobs

This quote sums up everything. The technological advancement is everywhere, and nursing is no different. Such online services like telehealth might help to automate many aspects of nursing.

With modern technology, patients can accomplish many facets of their own health care by accessing an online portal. They can also schedule appointments, see their test results, and request prescription refills. These virtual appointments facilitate them to see nurse practitioners or doctors via live video feed.

Likewise, chatbots can also assist patients with booking appointments and recapping them to take certain medications. You can think of any example you like. A likely scenario is one in which a chatbot nurse monitors health, give instructions and reminders to patients, and helps them find specialists in their area.

Bilingual Nurse Practitioners Will Be More Appreciated

The U.S. population has become increasingly diverse. As per the report by the U.S. Census Bureau, at least 350 different languages are spoken in American homes. Second to English, people speak Spanish in the United States. Around 40 million citizens speak Spanish at home.

So, considering the linguistic diversity of the country, bilingualism is valued more than ever. It is so appreciated that it will become a mandatory skill for nurse practitioners to have. It's a plus point for NPs who speak Spanish as their second language. So, I believe they will be more cherished in the future.

Nurses Will Choose To Specialize

Today, nurses are expected to specialize. This trend will also continue in the upcoming years. Nursing is a profession where there is an increased demand for higher levels of practice. The ones who choose to specialize are in higher demand and can often quote much higher salaries. Let me give you an example to explain this point. If LPNs have a salary of $44,240, RNs will quote the salary around $71,730. Considering this difference, many nurses will choose to specialize in the future.

The Ratio Of Male Nurse Practitioners Will Rise

Nursing is a female-dominated profession, but that is beginning to change. The American Association of Nursing Men continues to advocate for increasing the number of men in nursing programs throughout the United States.

Since 1960, there has been a visible trend in the number of male nurse practitioners continuing to rise. The proportion of male nurses rose from 2.2% in 1960 to 13% in 2015. As the stigma disappears, more and more men realize the benefits of the nursing profession. So, I expect the proportion of male nurses to increase further.

Focus Will Be Placed On Holistic Care

Holistic care is a way to achieve comprehensive care. The holistic nurse practitioners recognize the unique physical, psychological, emotional, spiritual, and environmental strengths of each patient. In addition to this, they can check the patient's weaknesses. The 'Patient Protection and Affordable Healthcare Act' focuses on providing patient-centered care.

In addition, one study published that new nurse practitioners and their patients can both benefit from holistic comfort theory. Hospitals and other medical institutions now emphasize a holistic approach in their delivery models.

Nurse Practitioners Will Become More Technology Savvy

Technology has always existed in the modern healthcare world. The nurse practitioners who are unfamiliar with the technology may get left behind. Today, NPs use a variety of technology-driven approaches to streamline their work. It includes electronic health records that track health history and smart beds that optimize patient placement.

According to the special report by *American Nurse Today*, technology offers many benefits. The benefits are strongly interwoven with quality care, patient satisfaction, and safety of the patients. Such technological innovation will be a part of the nursing profession. So, NPs will have to become more comfortable and confident with technological advancements.

The Health Informatics Will Become More Conventional

In response to the influx of healthcare technology, a new field has emerged: *Health Informatics*. This evolutionary capability uses data collected by information technology systems to create a more collaborative environment between patients and their various healthcare providers.

In 2015, a survey conducted by the Healthcare Information and Management Systems Society found significance in patient's quality care. The respondents of the study reported a positive impact on the quality of care patients received. The work of informatics nurses can achieve this goal. I believe that with higher average salaries and excellent job prospects, this field will generate more interest in the upcoming years.

Patients Will Become More Educated

In the age of smart devices, people are consuming more information than ever. They are well-informed about everything, and the nursing profession is no exception. Today, people have become more aware of their health-related statistics. However, it becomes quite worrying because they start self-medicating. But, looking at the positive side, people have become more educated. Nurse practitioners can now expect to see patients who have studied their symptoms or conditions online. They can also hope to see patients having a good understanding of their medications. Now, people have become more familiar with medicines best for them. The advertisements have made them smart enough to differentiate between good or bad.

So, healthcare professionals, especially NPs, must prepare themselves to deal with such educated patients. They can fix this by listening to patients' observations about their health and combining this information with their expertise and knowledge.

More Retail Clinics Will Open Up

Retail health clinics are not planned to address major issues. Instead, smaller healthcare services can be offered for patient's convenience. The retail clinics were looked upon as a disruption to healthcare industries. However, they provide an alternative channel for primary care. Also, these clinics are open seven days a week and don't require any appointments. This facility makes it more convenient for patients to just walk in and get the treatment.

The line between healthcare industries and retail clinics is fading. By 2025, the retail health clinic market is expected to reach $ 7.3 billion, with a compound annual growth rate (CAGR) of 20.3%. It is good news for nurse practitioners because many NPs have chosen to open their clinics in such retail locations.

Nursing Faculty Will Become More Captivating

The demand for RNs is undoubtedly growing. Paradoxically, many institutions have been forced to turn down qualified applicants because of the nursing faculty shortage. In 2016, a report on Enrollment and Graduations in Baccalaureate and Graduate Programs in Nursing was presented by (AACN).

It argued that the U.S. nursing schools have turned away 64,000 qualified applicants from baccalaureate and graduate nursing programs. The AACN identified budget constraints, an aging faculty, and increasing job competition as contributing factors to the faculty shortage. In response to the shortage, many initiatives have already been taken to make the faculty positions more attractive. The Jonas Nurse Leader Scholar Program is an example of such an initiative.

The program provides financial support to more than 1,000 scholars in 50 states across the United States. The program also aims to expand access to nursing departments in the future.

The Demand For Geriatric Nurse Practitioners Will Increase

Geriatrics is a medical field that covers older people's care. Geriatric nurse practitioners are the most critical professionals in this field because they often provide daily care for patients with special needs. The demand for such nurses has dramatically improved with the increased life expectancy in the country.

The Congressional Budget Office computes that by 2050, one-fifth of the U.S. population will be 65 or older. However, a 2016 paper by the National Academy of Medicine stated: *"Less than 1% of registered nurses and less than 3% of senior registered nurses have certifications in geriatrics."*

In the future, I am quite confident that more geriatric nurse practitioners will be required. They will naturally be required to take care of the aging population of baby boomers. For all the new nurse practitioners, who have recently joined the industry, I recommend you to go for geriatric certifications. With these certifications, you will be at the forefront of this highly sought-after specialty.

More Attention Will Be Given To Common Issues

Nursing is a gratifying profession, but like any other job, it has some challenges. A recent survey to identify these challenges was conducted by 'American Nurse Today.' In the study, 55% of respondents reported verbal abuse from patients. Besides, 36% stated that other employees or healthcare workers had verbally abused them.

Nurse practitioners experience compassion fatigue, also known as Secondary Traumatic Stress. This problem can manifest itself in higher rates of apathy, absenteeism, and mental and physical exhaustion.

Hospitals and other facilities have started giving the required attention to this problem. People are shifting their focus to them. In response, many organizations are beginning to emphasize the importance of self-care in protecting nurse practitioners from work-related stress.

Job Extension

The United States is indeed facing a shortage of nursing care. However, the crisis has not been as severe as many analysts predicted. This is because older nurses have delayed their retirement age. A 2014 Health Affairs study found that older nurses are still working in the field. The report found that 74% of nurses are still working at the age of 62, and 24% of nurses at the age of 69.

I expect this trend to continue in the upcoming years as well. However, there will be many job opportunities for the new entrants, but such opportunities will be limited to the hospital environment. With age, older nurses tend to move to non-hospital settings.

Skilled Nursing Facilities (Snfs) Will Diversify

Despite the aging population, SNFs have seen a consistent decline in occupancy numbers. The recent Health Dimensions Group noted that last year's occupancy rate fell from 82% to 79%. Because of this trend, SNP providers might start to add more services than just skilled nursing. Perhaps these services include home care, health care, and adult day care services, or behavioral services.

A good example of behavioral services includes people with substance abuse issues. Therefore, SNF nurses are expected to treat a variety of patients in the upcoming years.

Value-Based Care Will Be Trending

Value-based care consists of payment models based on value, not on volume. Many insurance companies are shifting from an output-based pay policy to a value-based pay policy. This transition came into existence after the Patient Protection and Affordable Care Act of 2010. Value-based care also provides a positive patient experience. In my opinion, it's a much more essential measure for healthcare providers than output-based care.

Nursing information specialists play an essential role in evaluating and reporting outcomes used in value-based billing models. Some healthcare providers have publicly indicated their patients' experience on their websites. So, I expect to see this change in the upcoming years as well.

Nurse Practitioners Will Support Greater Inclusions On Boards

Nurse practitioners are an integral part of each hospital's leadership team. Sadly, they are severely under-represented on most hospital board. In 2011s, The Institute of Medicine's "Nursing Futures" report found that 20% of hospital board members are doctors, and only 6% are nurses.

In response, the federation of the Board of Nurses was established in 2020. The federation had a goal of bringing 10,000 nurses to the board. This initiative was backed by the Robert Wood Johnson Foundation and the AARP. As of January 2020, the federation has more than 7,026 nurses on the hospitals' board of directors. Despite major progress, I expect this trend to continue in the upcoming years. However, the goal of 10,000 nurses is unlikely to be achieved by the end of this year.

Nurse Practitioners Will Become More Active In Battling The Opioid Crisis

The United States is in the midst of an opioid crisis. According to data from the National Institute of Drug Abuse, more than 115 people die from overdosing. The recent Patient and Community Support Act has taken many measures to help resolve the crisis. To truly end the epidemic, healthcare providers, including nurse practitioners, will need to play a more active role.

Opioid abuse begins with prescription drugs. The Lippincott Nursing Center has identified several ways where nurse practitioners can help in this problem. The solution includes addressing the crisis through responsible pain management practices. Besides, some methods support sensible opioid prescriptions, educating patients, and using non-opioid procedures to reduce the pain.

In terms of live-saving, the actions led by the nurse practitioners may be one of the essential health industry trends in upcoming years.

More Focus On Maternal Health

Since 1987, the pregnancy-related mortality rate has been doubled in the U.S. As per the statistics, the country was named the most dangerous place for a child's birth. This worrisome trend demanded a response from the health industry.

So, in 2018, the Senate approved Preventing Maternal Death Act with a winning consent. In the act, money was given to the states that can be used to review the cause of deaths. After investigation, it was found that some hospitals are not following the primary steps. In light of these shocking findings and government-funded initiatives, maternal health should continue to receive widespread attention in the upcoming years. I hope these implications make you understand the *Future of Nursing* in a better way. Nurse practitioners can prepare themselves well for the future with these points in mind.

As an NP, it is my responsibility to always look for new ways to improve. I believe nurse practitioners who embrace challenges, focus on professional development, and increase their knowledge, will secure excellent positions in the future. These findings can help you achieve a better job position in the upcoming years.

The nursing profession is indeed heading in the right direction. The World Health Organization (WHO) has declared this year as a *"Year of Nurse and Midwife."* It was entirely out of the blue to expect a year full of an international health crisis.

Today, where the entire nation is grappling with the impact of the virus, nurse practitioners, along with other health professionals, are fighting at the frontline. I must say that it's a perfect time to join the nursing industry. It's a time to show that we are all united against the pandemic crisis. As a Nurse Practitioner, I feel quite proud that nurses are offering healthcare services in every part of the world. Pompously, I can say that the nursing profession is in safe hands. Nursing is an ever-changing profession. It is one of the most sacred professions in the world. We see human beings in their challenging times.

It is our job to provide them healthcare services at their lowest times. Our job is to make their lives healthier and more enjoyable. I can certainly say that the profession is full of options, and multiple job opportunities are available for new graduates.

From the challenges of the first year to future implications, I have given my best to enlighten my readers. I wanted to share with the world that being an NP is not an easy profession, especially when you are fulfilling the medical treatment responsibilities of patients with various illnesses at once.

Moreover, working with multiple supervising physicians can be a considerable challenge. They all have varying styles of practice and attitudes toward medicine and treatments. It can be quite challenging to accommodate each physician's preferences.

Another big challenge that NPs face is the unconventional work schedule. Although it is quite flexible, it has its downside. In addition to day shifts, when working in the ER, you must also work a fair share of nights, evenings, weekends, and even holidays. For instance, it is challenging to work on Thanksgiving when the rest of your family is together, hosting a party. A flexible work schedule certainly comes with some sacrifice.

However, the biggest challenge of all will always be the expectations others have from you. You are expected to know as much as a physician, for instance, but with much less training and schooling. You become proficient with time, and you continually learn throughout your career. I believe this is both a positive and negative aspect of the nurse practitioner's career.

On the one hand, it ensures that your workday is never dull. The challenge of learning makes an NP's job intellectually stimulating and fulfilling. On the other hand, it can be frustrating and time-consuming to look up information and ask questions to your supervisors on a daily basis. These are a few of the many challenges I faced during my journey. I know that many other nurse practitioners also face similar issues in the profession. However, being able to serve others is the best feeling in the world, especially when you have nearly the same responsibilities for managing patients as a fully qualified doctor. To all the fresh nurse practitioners, the practical world is never going to be easy. Still, I hope my book proves to be a step by step guide for new graduates.

SHANE D GRINDLE

Made in the USA
Columbia, SC
12 January 2021